BABY MAKING FOR EVERYBODY

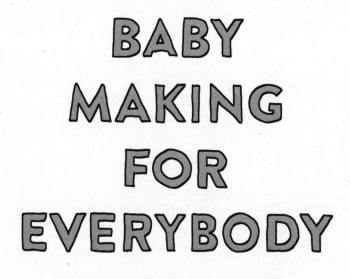

BABY MAKING FOR EVERYBODY

Family Building and Fertility for LGBTQ+ and Solo Parents

Ray Rachlin, LM, CPM
Marea Goodman, LM, CPM

balance

New York   Boston

Balance
Hachette Book Group
1290 Avenue of the Americas, New York, NY 10104
GCP-Balance.com
twitter.com/GCPBalance
instagram.com/GCPBalance

First Edition: April 2023

Balance is an imprint of Grand Central Publishing. The Balance name and logo are trademarks of Hachette Book Group, Inc.

The publisher is not responsible for websites (or their content) that are not owned by the publisher.

Balance books may be purchased in bulk for business, educational, or promotional use. For information, please contact your local bookseller or the Hachette Book Group Special Markets Department at special.markets@hbgusa.com.

Library of Congress Cataloging-in-Publication Data
Names: Rachlin, Ray, author. | Goodman, Marea, author.
Title: Baby making for everybody : family building and fertility for LGBTQ+ and solo parents / Ray Rachlin, LM, CPM, Marea Goodman, LM, CPM.
Description: First edition. | New York : Balance, 2023. | Includes bibliographical references and index.
Identifiers: LCCN 2022047952 | ISBN 9781538725863 (trade paperback) | ISBN 9781538725870 (ebook)
Subjects: LCSH: Human reproductive technology—Popular works. | Pregnancy—Popular works. | Human reproduction—Popular works. | Sexual minority parents. | Same-sex parents. | Sexual minorities' families.
Classification: LCC RG133.5 .R33 2023 | DDC 618.30086/64—dc23/eng/20221114
LC record available at https://lccn.loc.gov/2022047952

ISBNs: 9781538725863 (trade paperback), 9781538725870 (ebook)

Printed in the United States of America

LSC-C

Printing 1, 2023

To all the queer midwives, organizers, and agitators who came before me. Thank you for teaching me how to be an activist, calling me in, and showing me a future where liberation is possible.

To Asher, thank you for unwavering love and support, for always challenging me to be better, and for building a family with me.

To my baby. Your long journey into our family has taught me so much as a baba and a midwife. Thank you for choosing us to be your parents.

To my midwifery partner, Victoria. Without your partnership, friendship, and shared call schedule this book would not be possible. Thank you for midwifing with me ☺

To my clients, thank you for allowing me to walk alongside you in your journey to parenthood. It is the greatest honor.

—Ray

To my kids: Thank you for making me a mama, for all the cuddles and growth opportunities. I love being your parent.

To Andrea: Thank you for introducing me to fertility care, doing life with me, and inviting me into parenthood with you. It's the greatest honor and joy.

To all my clients and midwifery teachers: I'm forever grateful to have learned from you and by your sides.

—Marea

Contents

Who We Are and Why We Midwife

First off, we are so excited that you're reading this book! It has truly been a labor of love for both Ray and Marea, two millennial midwives who have dedicated their professional (and much of their personal) lives to the project of queer and nontraditional family building and parenthood. We both envision a world where there are tons of thriving, interconnected LGBTQ+ and solo parents,* where everybody has access to all the information and support they need to create and grow families in the ways that make the most sense for them. We wrote this book with that vision in mind.

If you've picked up this book, you are likely in the midst of your journey of building your family as an LGBTQ+ and/or solo parent. We know that building family outside the traditional heterosexual, nuclear family model is a huge project, one that comes with many (and we mean many!) questions and things to consider. From finding sperm, eggs, and/or a uterus, to understanding your unique fertility picture, to all the legal considerations, and more—building your LGBTQ+ and/or solo parent family can be a complex process. Whether you are just in the beginning stages of exploring all your possible paths forward or you have a clear picture of your next steps, we've got you covered.

---

* Note: Almost all resources for hopeful solo parents use the language *single mother by choice*. We've chosen not to use this phrase because (a) it is not gender-inclusive, and (b) it implies that people who chose single parenthood are superior to people who became single parents by circumstance.

The idea for this book was conceived when Marea was newly pregnant for the first time (with her third child) after going through the IUI process, and Ray had recently finalized their donor and begun their own conception journey. Experiencing queer fertility as people, not as midwives guiding others through this process, made us realize how needed this book really is.

What we're writing about isn't new: It's what queer people and solo parents have been figuring out around how to become parents for generations. Without models, books, or systems to support us, we have relied on our resilience and community wisdom to guide our paths forward. This book is our next step in passing on our community's collective knowledge, and an opportunity to lift up all the ways our families creatively come together to grow and nourish the next generation.

Anyone who wants a baby but lacks sperm or eggs knows that the conception journey starts long before a positive pregnancy test. Our hope for this book is that it's not only a guide to building LGBTQ+, solo parent, and other radical families but also a celebration of the amazing families our communities create.

In the following chapters, we will walk you through all the information you need to navigate fertility and family building. We will talk about finding sperm and egg donors, surrogacy, understanding and tracking fertility, and the different insemination options available to create a pregnancy. We'll discuss how transgender people can use their genetic material to become parents and use their body to feed their baby (should they wish to). We will also explore the worlds of fostering and adoption, the steps to take to become a foster or adoptive parent, and how families prepare to parent children in crisis.

Then we talk about early pregnancy, and navigating miscarriage and infertility as queer people and solo parents. We'll guide you through the legal components of family formation for LGBTQ+, solo, and poly families, as well as discuss how to talk about your family-building plans with your family of origin and how to line up support for yourself in the postpartum or post-adoption period and beyond.

Throughout the book, you'll find practical information about your options for having children and how to make decisions within the systems that are not designed to meet the needs of LGBTQ+ people and folks pursuing solo parenthood. You'll also find many personal stories from people just like you, who grew their families and were generous enough to share their experiences with us.

And for good measure, you'll find an appendix of resources and templates to assist you on your journey to parenthood at the end of this book. You can also visit our website, www.babymakingforevery body.com, for more regularly updated information about resources and support groups, as well as inspiring stories from other LGBTQ+ and solo parents.

We hope that this book helps you feel prepared to embark on your own family-making journey and connects you to the growing community of other LGBTQ+ and solo parents who are paving the way for more and more families like ours.

———————

Like many millennial midwives, we met on Instagram. There aren't a ton of openly queer midwives, especially in the home birth world, and even fewer that provide fertility care and inseminations or that center the needs of LGBTQ+ families. Marea's practice, Restore Midwifery, was originally founded in Oakland, California, and now operates in Santa Cruz. Ray's practice, Refuge Midwifery, is based in Philadelphia, Pennsylvania. As of this publication, we have collectively been practicing community midwives for nearly fifteen years. Together we have provided hundreds of IUIs and spent countless hours counseling people through the sometimes-dizzying processes of choosing a sperm donor, tracking ovulation, timing inseminations, and deciding upon the next steps if the IUI process doesn't seem to be working.

In 2020, each of us had the idea separately to begin an anthology project of LGBTQ+ conception stories as a way to connect to and educate our communities around their family-building options. After that first conversation when we discovered how aligned our visions were for supporting our communities in the project of family building, we knew we had to team up. Our idea evolved from story sharing into a how-to guide for all things LGBTQ+ and solo parent family building, and this book was conceived.

Marea

I am an Ashkenazi-Jewish queer mom/mommy/occasional dad, living on unceded Awaswas / Amah Mutsun territory aka Santa Cruz, California. I grew up with many privileges that have supported me to write this book, including class privilege, white privilege, and the privilege of having my queerness fully accepted by my family of origin.

I started attending births as a doula in 2011 and graduated from UC Berkeley in 2012. Soon after my first experiences of hospital births, I decided to start apprenticing as a home birth midwife. Supporting people to birth in a safe and supported way in their own homes was the first thing I'd found that felt completely in line with my feminist, anti-racist, body-autonomy values.

I got licensed as a midwife by the California Medical Board in 2015, then worked at birth centers in El Paso, Texas, and Ciudad Vieja, Guatemala. In 2016, I founded my home birth practice, Restore Midwifery, in Oakland, California. The next year, I started dating Andrea, my now-wife, who at the time had a six-year-old-daughter and had recently conceived a baby as a planned solo parent by choice. She taught me how to provide inseminations, and thanks to her I incorporated queer fertility support into my practice. Three years later, I started my own conception process, and our blended family got bigger.

It was surreal to experience firsthand the emotions that I've counseled my clients through for years—the doubts and anxieties surrounding ideal insemination timing and the curious mixture of joy and shock at seeing my first positive pregnancy test. Seeing PREGNANT on the Clearblue pregnancy test exactly two weeks after my first insemination felt like a dream. After the shock wore off, I cried overwhelmed tears, then happy ones, and then called my parents and two best friends to share the news. My partner, our two kids, and I took a selfie in the bathroom while the two-year-old clutched the positive pregnancy test in their little hands.

When I started bleeding the next day, I didn't expect to feel so heartbroken. I knew that almost one-third of all pregnancies end in miscarriage. I was aware of the prevalence of what's known as a "chemical pregnancy." I had supported many friends and clients through the painful process of passing their pregnancies at home and sat with them afterward, holding their hands, handing them tissues. But I'd never known that sense of emptiness within my own body. Even after knowing I was pregnant for only twenty-four hours, the intensity of losing my potential baby was devastating, made more intense because I questioned the validity of grieving a chemical pregnancy.

For me, this has been the theme of becoming pregnant for the first time after spending almost a decade as a reproductive health provider: I didn't really get it until it happened in my own body. And yet, through my own roller coaster of conception, I felt accompanied by all the people I'd known going through their own ups and downs. When I got pregnant again on my second insemination, I remembered what I'd heard another midwife tell a shared client during the first trimester of her second pregnancy: "You're never quite as confident about a pregnancy after having a miscarriage." Her words resonated in my mind every time I glanced at the toilet paper after going to the bathroom, fearing, and almost expecting, to see it tinged with blood.

I didn't think I would be an anxious pregnant person. As a home birth midwife, I deeply believe that our bodies are capable, amazing things—adept at producing life (when we choose to). But there were many moments during that first trimester when I didn't feel that my body and my baby were okay. My partner, who had birthed our two children and is also a midwife, had to talk me down from that anxiety ledge at least once a week. During those moments, it helped to remember all my friends and clients who had gone through similar experiences and come out the other side.

I share this with you because it is the foundation of my desire to write this book. Namely, that family building is too often something that happens in private, without the necessary support and hand-holding from close community. For queer and prospective solo parents, the extra hurdles many of us face in having children are almost never reflected in mainstream culture. Many people have no idea how much a single vial of sperm costs from a bank (hint: It's about one hundred times more expensive than you'd expect), or how upsetting it feels for some people not to be able to make a baby that shares their and their partner's DNA.

Personal narratives, when shared, hold the potential to help other people feel less alone in their process. My hope is that these stories, and the practical information provided in these chapters, will help you feel supported and deeply empowered through your own profound and unique family-building journey.

Ray

I am a white, nonbinary femme, second-generation, queer Jewish midwife, new baba, living on the unceded Lenape land of

Philadelphia. I was raised by an amazing single mom in New York and grew up poor. I went to Queens College (at the same time as my mom) and became an activist. Activism in the other labor movement landed me in a doula training in 2010, and three years into doula-ing I made the leap to midwifery school in Oregon in 2013. I graduated and passed NARM (the certification exam for direct entry midwives) in 2016. One year later I moved across the country to Philly and launched my practice, Refuge Midwifery, with the hope of being a resource for LGBTQ+ families and bridging access to the midwifery model of care through community education, fertility, home IUI care, and home birth.

Less than a year into my practice, I had a few nonbinary and trans pregnant folks in my care. I asked them if they knew any other trans and gender-nonconforming folks who were pregnant or trying to be, and everyone said no. So, with a dozen or so queer clients in my practice (some pregnant, some in the process of trying to conceive), I sent out a Doodle poll for a potluck in the park.

Folks showed up, and it was a little awkward at first but also very sweet. So we did it again. And again. Pretty soon the potlucks outgrew the park and moved into different attendees' homes. We met every other month, and then we started a listserv because at the time there were no listservs for LGBTQ+ people trying to conceive or LGBTQ+ pregnant people in this area. Some of my clients became friends outside the potlucks, and about a year later we opened up to folks outside my practice as well.

The last few gatherings before the COVID-19 pandemic occurred in packed homes with so many snacks, questions about sperm, and a few pregnant bellies and babies conceived through IUI. It was a reminder of how resilient our communities are. Wherever we are left out, we create our own resources within our communities.

I sometimes joked at the potlucks that I was organizing all of this to have a queer-parent community for when I was finally ready to try to conceive. Everyone in the group had heard our harrowing sperm journey of asking my partner's brother to be our donor and subsequently being denied ten months later. We had asked our second potential known donor a few weeks before the pandemic shut everything down, so I never got to directly update the only people in my life who understood how incredibly long and arduous queer conception can sometimes be with my family-building plans.

By the time my partner and I actually started trying to conceive at the end of 2020, I felt like we had been trying to get pregnant for years. I was surprised by how anxiety producing every aspect of cycle tracking was, and being an expert in queer conception felt absolutely useless. I wanted to talk about *all* of it with everyone I could connect with, but I wasn't sure if I was oversharing and being inappropriate. Heterosexual norms around conception and early pregnancy felt more stifling than ever, and I didn't know how to strike a balance between finding the support I needed and protecting myself emotionally.

While launching into my own baby-making journey, I was also co-launching a trans-competent fertility and birth directory with an accompanying queer-conception-stories blog the same month Marea launched a queer-parenting anthology book project. Once we discovered that we were conceiving very similar family-planning resources for the LGBTQ+ community, we knew we needed to team up.

———————

Where society and systems fail to meet our needs, our queer community nurtures us and shows us the way. When we see other LGBTQ+ and/or solo parents having children and growing their families, and when we share with one another what we know, each individual benefits from the collective knowledge and the examples that our community sets.

This book is for the young queer couple curious about how they can someday become moms. It's for the hopeful solo parent who is craving to see themselves and their family reflected in our culture. It's for the gay dads figuring out how they are going to build their family. It's for poly families who have yet to see a resource that includes them. And it's for the teenage trans kid who heard from their doctor that by beginning hormone-replacement therapy, they are sacrificing their future fertility (they aren't). This book is for all of you.

As midwives, we are experts in uteruses and the people who have them. This book will be a guide to conception for all the folks who lack sperm in creating their family, and it will be a jumping-off point for folks looking for eggs and uteruses to find their pathway to creating a family, as well as those building their families through fostering and adoption.

We are both born and raised in the United States and we continue to work in the US. For this reason, much of this information, particularly information around legal considerations, is specific to this country. However, the information we include about fertility, inseminations, miscarriage, and infertility, as well as some of the social/ emotional aspects, is applicable to people living all over the world.

We both envision a world where there are tons of thriving, interconnected solo and LGBTQ+ parents, where everybody has access to all the information and support they need to create and grow families in the ways that make the most sense for them. We are so excited to support you in this journey, and we hope that you will find the information, care, and community wisdom you need on these pages. It is our deepest hope that this book can be an extension of the radical family-building community—and that it can accompany, support, and nourish you through your own complicated, messy, glorious process of growing your family.

Let's get started.

CHAPTER 1

Why Do You Want to Be a Parent, Anyway?

> Having a family with kids was something I always knew I wanted. I loved the idea of parenting and what that meant. I was constantly asking myself: What were the skills, experiences, tools, that I would bring to this parenting role and relationship? My partner and I wanted to build a family *our* way and raise a young person to be free and fierce and kind and to love soil and birds. Someone who would grow up thinking critically and expansively about gender and race and their place in the world. —Danny Alvarez

We've found through both our midwifery practices and our own experiences that during the process of growing a family as LGBTQ+ or solo people, folks can sometimes get bogged down in the details of the *how* and lose touch with the *why*. This makes sense to us—after all, the *how* can be overwhelming, with many steps, new decisions, and costs to consider. One minute you're imagining holding your future child in your arms and the next you're doom-scrolling through donor profiles, peeing on sticks, crunching the numbers (again) to see if you can eke out another round of IUI or wondering how in the h*ll you can afford IVF. Add in all the emotions and it's no wonder so many of us can lose sight of the forest for the trees.

We know it can be stressful. We've counseled hundreds of people through this process, and we've been there ourselves. That's why we want to start this book by supporting you to get in touch with your deep desires, hopes, dreams, and intentions around parenting before you embark on the logistics of actually making that happen. By starting this way, we hope you can feel resourced and supported, and that you can carry these feelings with you throughout your family-building journey.

Why Do People Choose to Become Parents, and How Do They Prepare?

Before we dive into why *you* want to be a parent, let's acknowledge that queer people and single people have always been parents. Generations before us have found ways to start and nurture our families, to find community, and to thrive. We also have faced tremendous adversity. Social stigma and lack of resources have trapped many single mothers in the margins of society for generations.[1] In the 1970s and 1980s, almost all lesbian mothers who fought for custody of their children in court lost, and it wasn't until 1997 that New Jersey became the first state in the US to allow gay couples to adopt a child together.[2]

In the years since Stonewall, LGBTQ+ rights have grown by leaps and bounds, and so have visibility and acceptance of our families. These days, 48 percent of LGBTQ+ millennials are planning on becoming parents,[3] and an estimated 2.7 million single-parent households chose solo parenthood.[4] Single and LGBTQ+ people are finding their ways to parenthood, but systems haven't caught up with the needs of our families yet.

As reproductive healthcare professionals, we deeply believe that every person deserves the right to decide whether or not they want to become parents, and how. Both of us have known that we wanted to become parents for a long time. Raising children offers a type of closeness that most of us have never experienced before. Babies and young children have profound stamina for intimacy—they want to be held and cuddled and played with constantly, consistently providing oxytocin and yumminess. For those of us who love personal growth (ahem—Marea), parenting may be the most effective path to enlightenment. You'll be forced to grow and heal in ways you hadn't imagined before having children. And besides, parenting is fun! As adults, we can sometimes get stuck in adulting, and it's helpful to have little people around us who are immensely thrilled when the trash truck comes around.

Parenting is also f*cking challenging. It can be exhausting—from the lack of sleep when you have a newborn to the particular form of mental exhaustion caused by playing imagination games for hours, parenting requires profound wells of energy and patience. If you're in a partnership, becoming a parent can put immense stress on relationships, changing dynamics and drastically decreasing the amount of time you spend having romantic time with your significant other. The demand that parenting puts on financial resources is profound, and for many families, the expenses start to pile up even before a child is conceived.

Agh! But It's *So Annoying* Not to Be Able to Accidentally Make a Baby!

Trust us—we know. But maybe this is a blessing in disguise? As LGBTQ+ and solo people, often we are *required* to bring tons of intention into our journey to parenting. Although it can be complicated and costly to figure out how we want to grow our families, the care we bring to our family-building journeys can deeply support our mental, emotional, spiritual, and physical well-being. Our children benefit from the knowledge that we worked hard to invite them into our families—that love is a powerful feeling for a child to have.

Because biology, medical transition, or relationship status

necessitates that we plan and prepare for every aspect of our family expansion, we have the opportunity to think through many important aspects of the life-changing process of becoming a parent. This preparation can simultaneously heighten the best parts of parenting and create more ease around the challenging ones. For example, we can start saving money for donor sperm or eggs or insemination support, gather hand-me-down baby supplies from friends or people giving their baby stuff away on Craigslist, or move into a co-op house with people interested in supporting us with childcare. And we can find an awesome therapist whom we trust enough to heal some of our childhood trauma so we don't unconsciously act it out on our children.

> When we started talking about having kids, some conversations made us scared about how much work our relationship required in order to feel ready. And then we went to therapy. And we committed and recommitted to working on us because we both felt growth from it and in that time, we learned how to communicate with each other. I always knew I wanted a big family but there was work I needed to do to get there. I started reparenting myself in ways I needed and letting my partner help, too. We learned about co-regulating, which feels like a very queer and ecological form of intimacy. —Joe Lehrman

We don't believe that it's possible to be fully prepared for all the changes that becoming a parent will bring into your life. The intensity of the emotions of having a child, not to mention the unprecedented demands on your time and attention, means that no person can truly know what it's like until they experience it themselves. However, we can prepare ourselves by proactively working on our own childhood wounds and past trauma, practicing accessing inner resources for holding all the unknowns of pre-conception and parenting, bringing in our community, and lining up all the support we can. It can make a difference to our experiences of the whole family-building process.

I'm a single mom by choice, which means that from the beginning I had to plan my choices. Before I became a parent, my parents agreed to watch my kid three mornings a week so that I could continue my job as a community college professor. I secured a babysitter, backup babysitter, backup backup babysitter. I made a financial plan—a rough plan, but a plan nonetheless. I read all the big books about parenting and the thin ones as well, got hand-me-down clothing and toys from six generous friends, took parenting classes, and moved a hard-to-disassemble crib from the spare room to my bedroom and back again. Even the pregnancy itself was planned through careful monitoring at a reproductive endocrinologist's office. The first indication that parenting requires flexibility that I might not be able to handle was the day I learned that I was not having one baby but two—a two-for-one special, my nurse said. —Elizabeth Catanese

Of course, even the best-laid plans can get uprooted. With all this talk about being intentional, we also know that we can't control many parts of this process. While we encourage you to take the time to understand the road map ahead, we also want to invite you to bring as much flexibility and gentleness to this process as possible.

Knowing your own *why* is what will allow you to approach this process with compassion and clarity, and in the following pages we hope you'll find guidance, community wisdom, and some questions to ponder that can leave you feeling clearer on why you want to become a parent, as well as any areas that you're interested in growing before embarking on parenthood.

Why Do *You* Want to Become a Parent?

Let's start with this question: Why do you want to become a parent? Some people may feel that they want a child to connect to a greater purpose in life. Others are looking for a certain kind of closeness and connection that only a child can provide. For others, they imagine that sharing a baby with their partner will connect them together forever, and this can be a primary motive in family formation. Without judgment, it's important to spend some time reflecting on this huge decision to bring another life into the world or to create a new family with a child who was born into another family.

WHAT'S YOUR WHY?

The following questions are to encourage you to explore your *why* about pursuing parenthood. We recommend spending some time journaling about each of them. (Try to do so without thinking about your answers too hard, just letting the words come.) Afterward, if you have a partner or a prospective co-parent, these can become great conversation prompts. As with all offerings throughout this book, feel free to alter these prompts in any way and make them your own.

When I imagine becoming a parent, I feel...

I realized I wanted to become a parent when...

I want / don't want to have a biological child because... (circle one, and explain)

If I don't have a child, I would feel...

I'm scared that in becoming a parent, I will...

I'm excited to become a parent because... .

I will know I'm ready to parent when...

I will know that I have enough community support to parent when...

Getting in Touch with Your Priorities

After answering these questions, take some time to determine your top three reasons for becoming a parent. Write them down on a piece of paper and keep it somewhere visible—you can tape it to your wall in your bedroom or keep it somewhere that you'll be able to see throughout the coming months or years of building your family.

This may look something like:

MY FAMILY-BUILDING PRIORITIES

To raise a child with as much patience, tenderness, and love as I possibly can.

To have a child who is genetically related to me.

To heal generational trauma through parenting.

Your priorities may look very different from this. But we think it's helpful to create a visual that can serve as your guiding light in this process of family building. Remember, you can always change or revise your priorities. Flexibility, a key to parenthood, is also essential for conception.

As you read this book, we also encourage you to think about your needs in *how* you build your family. What, of the help available for conception or family building, resonates best with your lived experience and family-planning wishes? Thinking about your experiences with medical systems, family, and your own body up until this point, you may consider questions like:

- Have your experiences receiving healthcare felt comfortable or uncomfortable?
- Do you want to lead your conception process, have a medical professional lead your process, or something in between?
- Do you want lots of information about your body's fertility from medical tests? What is your initial reaction to the idea of fertility treatments?
- Is privacy or relationships—with partner(s) or donors—a priority for you?
- How do you define family? Is being biologically related to your child important to you? Why or why not?
- Are there ways you do or don't want a child to come into your family?

There is no one-size-fits-all approach to the tools we use to grow our families. Understanding our priorities in how we want to navigate care and the whole conception process can help us be empowered regardless of how our path to parenthood unfolds.

I was always very clear that I wanted to lead my fertility process. I knew when I was ovulating and I wanted the least amount of intervention from doctors possible because I had not had positive experiences receiving healthcare. That priority guided me and my partner through a lot of decision-making, through switching donors and conception methods, and later when I decided to pursue infertility interventions I used my primary care doctor who I trusted instead of a fertility clinic. My conception journey was longer than I anticipated, but I felt in control and my partner and I had the time and space to make decisions that were right for us. —Ray

So What Can I Plan For?

Whether you're planning to build your family through your own or your partner's pregnancy, a surrogate, or fostering and adoption, preparing to talk about your child's origin story will be emotionally supportive for your children and your family as a whole. It's also very helpful to plan for practical support, both logistically and emotionally. In a larger system that doesn't always validate LGBTQ+ and solo parents, knowing the internal and external resources to lean on will help you, your partner(s), and also your future kids weather the challenges that lie ahead. Some of the considerations you can plan for are your kid's experiences, the relationship you'll have to your kid's biological family, your own family and community support, and how you'll address intergenerational trauma.

Putting Thought into Your Kid's Experiences About Having a Donor or a Surrogate

If you're planning to conceive with the help of donor eggs, sperm, or a surrogate, consider how you will talk to your future children about where they came from. We have had many clients choose known donors because they want their future children to be able to know the person who provided half of their genetic material as they grow. For families using anonymous donors, get clear on why this is the right path for your family and how you want to tell your children about where they came from.

Ray has had a handful of clients write and print conception books for their kids—compiling information about how their child was conceived with the help of donors or surrogates in children's book format. This offers kids an age-appropriate way to know where they came from, and how desired and loved they were even before they were conceived.

> We are very friendly with both of our children's surrogates. We have an open-door policy, which means that whenever they want to visit the kids, they can. We drove down to bring the kids to our second surrogate's daughter's seventh birthday, and our first surrogate came to our wedding. —Neill

Thinking About Adoption or Fostering and How to Relate to a Child's Biological Family

Whether you know now that you want to grow your family through fostering or adoption, or you come to the decision later in your family-building journey, it's important to consider how you want to relate to your child's biological family of origin and maintain a connection to their culture if it differs from yours. There is a ton of information about how important it is for an adopted child's experience to maintain connection with their biological family.[5] Preparing for this now, emotionally as well as logistically, will impact your future child(ren)'s emotional well-being. (We'll talk about this more in chapter 6.)

Family and Community Support

When our family-formation journey starts long before the first pregnancy test, we have more time to gather our network to support our kids as they grow. As queer midwives, we know the power of chosen community and have seen how amazing it can be for kids to have so many close, loving grown-ups in their lives, whether they are biologically related or not. Community support also means you have more time and space to be an adult and care for yourself, and caring for yourself allows you to show up better as a parent. It's so good for the kids—not to mention *you*—to get community and family support on board as special people in your future children's lives, even before they come into being.

Preparing to Parent—Healing Generational Trauma

There's nothing like parenting to remind you that, like it or not, you are a product of your own parents, and they are a product of theirs. The moment that Marea became a parent, she started worrying about a thousand things a day: from her kids falling out a window to them getting scurvy from not eating enough fruits and vegetables. Many of her worries were ridiculous carbon copies of concerns her own parents had when she grew up. Now, five years later, Marea stands in front of the TV watching the Golden State Warriors exactly like her dad watched the Knicks while she was young.

Whether we are conscious of it or not, the way we parent is similar to how we were parented, unless we put the effort in to process and change it. It's so important that we take some time to reflect on our own childhoods, and take action to heal from the parts that didn't serve us, to avoid causing hurts to our children similar to what we experienced as young ones. Putting thought, intention, and healing into your own childhood wounds will do wonders in supporting your ability to kindly and compassionately parent your future children.

The following worksheet is meant to spark some of these conversations about family patterns. If you have a partner or partners, these questions can encourage dialogue between you with the hope of supporting you to start disentangling the web of childhood emotions *before* you have a child of your own to raise. If you or your partner(s) or potential co-parents had a painful or traumatic childhood, we recommend going through this section with a friend, therapist, or other support person. Trauma from our families of origin does have a tendency to come up when we pursue becoming parents ourselves.

THINGS YOU LIKED, AND DIDN'T LIKE, ABOUT HOW YOU WERE RAISED

Some of the best things my parent(s) or caregiver(s) did for me as a child were...

What lessons, experiences, or expectations that I learned from my parent(s) or caregiver(s) were harmful? What wouldn't I want to pass on to the next generation?

Who was an adult who supported me during my childhood, and what did they do that made me feel supported?

How safe, loved, and cared for was I as a child? How did my caregivers help me feel safe or unsafe?

When I'm a parent, I want to be the kind of parent who...

When I'm a parent, I want to be the kind of parent who doesn't...

It's most important to me that my child feels

_____.

When the World Is on Fire, How Do You Want to Parent?

When Marea was early in her pregnancy, she and her family were forced to spend most of five weeks indoors to avoid breathing as much of the noxious smoke caused by California's wildfire season as possible. It was a hard time for her—not only was it stressful to breathe poisonous air and to be trapped in a house with two antsy kids, but it was also scary thinking about the kind of world that this tiny baby who didn't yet even know how to breathe would inherit. What would the world look like for this child in ten years? In fifty?

We know that the way humans in the Global North are using resources is unsustainable, and climate change is leading many people to question if it's ethical to bring new humans into the world. Some people who want to parent are choosing to foster or adopt instead of creating a new human, and others who desire pregnancy or a genetically related child may grapple with the environmental costs of their decisions. There is no right answer to this question of whether or how to become parents because of climate change, but as midwives we know that the desire to create, birth, and parent children is one of the oldest truths of the human experience.

For all of us choosing to pursue parenthood, we must align ourselves to fight against the racist, capitalist system that's creating the climate crisis and set an example for our children, who will grow up needing to care for our planet in new ways. Becoming parents has the potential to help us feel more connected to our planet and what it needs for us to continue to live here. We can educate ourselves and organize for change with the intention of taking care of our children, grandchildren, and great-grandchildren, as well as all of their extended communities.

The last weeks of October 2019 were sweltering. My family had just bought a farm, I was nine months' pregnant, and we were sitting pretty in a record-breaking heat wave. I had been in prodromal labor for three days and three nights. My doula told me to walk, so that's what my wife and I did.

We walked the farm in the evenings, after the sun dipped behind the trees, long shadows giving the illusion that things might be cooler. The average temperature was ninety-eight degrees with 90 percent humidity, and I was contracting every seven minutes on the dot. We walked past our small herd of Nigerian goats, big-bellied pregnant mamas panting in the shade of an old oak. These animals were bred for the heat and were still miserable. I had never empathized with an animal more.

Halloween brought relief via a stormy cold front and our son, Asher. We spent the fall and winter cozied up in front of a fire admiring our baby in total bliss, but the heat came back with a vengeance, and this year is even worse. It is not even July and we haven't dipped below ninety degrees in over a week. We play outside in the early morning but past 11:00 a.m., it's too dangerous to be outdoors.

I can't ignore the headlines I see on social media about melting glaciers and devastating floods in one region while another is being ravaged by never-ending fires, and Europe is being hit by tornadoes! I worry. A lot. Is it too late? Have we set our children up for failure on a dying planet? I hope not.

We are doing our best, teaching Asher a self-sustaining life, to utilize natural resources sparingly and only as needed. I have to hope that we are raising a child who will want better for our world and who will work with his generation to ensure a better future, not only for themselves but for generations to come. —Emily Krawczyk

We know that climate change is a huge topic, and it can be easier to try to tune it out than to actually engage in changing it. But we also know as parents and future parents (and humans in general) that we *need* to be working on making the planet livable to every human and animal on it. Perhaps we are a group of people uniquely positioned to make a difference in protecting our planet. Our kids need us to be.

> I don't know how we'll turn the tide on climate change or the many other injustices we face every day. I wonder if there is enough community love to fight against corporate greed, so that we can switch to clean energy. But I refuse to imagine a future for my son, and all children, that is not bright and beautiful. Our children deserve clean air, clean water, and clean soil. They deserve to see the complex ecosystems and all the species that inhabit them thrive on this rock we all call home. Our children deserve to thrive. —Cassie Walston

We know that there are important logistics to consider when embarking on our family-building journeys and that at times it can feel overwhelming. So we've included this decision tree as a tool to help guide you through navigating many of your potential decisions related to becoming a parent.

Now that we've put some thought into why we want to become parents, we are ready to talk about step one for folks pursuing biological parenthood—finding the gametes (aka sperm and eggs) you need!

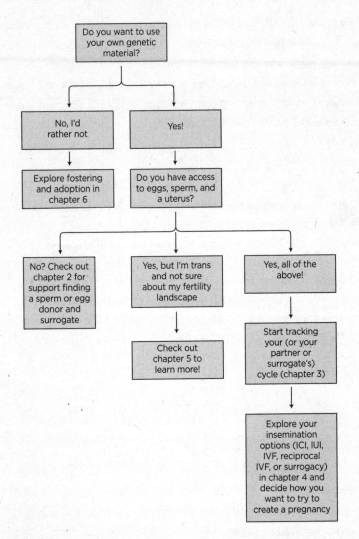

We're going to be diving into how to find sperm and egg donors as well as, for people without uteruses in their relationships, gestational carriers or surrogates. For those of you who are clear that you will be forming your families through fostering and adoption, feel free to skip to chapter 6.

CHAPTER 2

Sperm, Eggs, and Uteruses—Where to Get 'Em When You Need 'Em

There are three essential components that create a pregnancy: sperm, egg, and uterus. Some LGBTQ+ families have all the components to make a baby, but most do not. So the question is: When we lack one or two of those items, how do we go about getting them? Finding genetic material for your future children can be, to say the least, a roller coaster. Many of our clients spend months weighing the options, from buying sperm from a bank or traveling to a known donor (near or far!) for monthly inseminations to poring over sperm-bank websites and listening to voice recordings of potential donors. When people lack eggs or a uterus to grow a pregnancy, the prospects of how to make a baby can become even more daunting.

In this chapter we'll be talking about all the ways you can access donor sperm or eggs to create a baby, as well as how families find surrogates to grow their babies. We'll start with universal considerations for all people needing a donor, and then go into more detail about sperm donors on page 30, egg donors on page 41, and surrogacy on page 46.

As midwives and queer people who have gone through this process firsthand, we can definitively say there is no one-size-fits-all answer. Both of us had imagined ourselves using a local known donor and doing inseminations in our own homes with fresh sperm. And for both of us, COVID-19, being on-call as midwives, and some of the very human logistics of using a known donor took us down the path of IUI with banked sperm.

We recommend approaching your search for a donor with a grain of salt. Choosing a donor is important, yes. But having a child is the goal, and the donor is just one of the steps to getting there. You can change your *how* without compromising your *why* (take a quick look at the note you wrote yourself in chapter 1 as many times as you need to), and we encourage you to be open to changing plans. When you're running around after a two-year-old trying to get them to put on their pants, you won't be thinking about where you got their genetic material.

Through my three-plus years of trying to conceive, I got a no from the first two known donors I asked, and then tried with two other known donors. I spent months flying to Portland, Oregon, and it was so stressful that I made a no-flying-for-sperm rule. Years before starting my TTC process, I had scoured the banks for mixed-race (East Asian and white) donors and hadn't felt connected to the three donors who came up. After trying with my known donors, I decided to look at one bank that friends had recommended and found a donor that felt right. I didn't hesitate and bought the vial within thirty minutes of sitting down at my computer! That month, I tried with my known donor as well as the vial from the sperm bank and I got pregnant. When my baby was three months old, we did a DNA test along with my known donor and found out this kiddo's DNA came from the sperm bank.
—Alison Lin

WHAT ARE GAMETES?

Gametes are single-chromosome (haploid) sex cells, like sperm or egg cells, that are able to unite with another sex cell to create a double-chromosome (diploid) individual. When we say gametes, we're talking about an individual's sperm or eggs.

UNIVERSAL CONSIDERATIONS

How to Choose a Donor: Centering Your Priorities

Later in this chapter, we talk in depth about all the things related to donors—how sperm and egg donation works, the differences between known and anonymous donors, and all the logistics involved in how to make a baby using your donor's genetic material. But first, let's talk about your priorities in finding a donor. Getting clear on what qualities you would like in a donor is one of the first major steps in your family-building journey. There are many, many qualities people look for, and people's priorities range from "I literally just want sperm or eggs that will help me conceive" to "I'm looking for a donor who matches my partner's ethnicity, height, eye color, and education status *exactly*." We encourage you to be honest with yourself about what is important to you. This is the time to be candid about your needs, approach your own desires without judgment, and remember that change is possible—getting clear on your priorities is only one part of how you'll make your donor decision.

The following table is meant to support you in beginning this soul-searching process. We've filled in some of the popular characteristics many of our clients and friends search for in donors, and we recommend that you fill this table out with as many potential donor qualities as possible. These ideal donor qualities can help inform your choice between a known and an anonymous donor (more on this soon), as well as help you choose from the many donor options at a sperm or egg bank.

Ideal Donor Qualities

- Kindness
- Looks/attractiveness
- Similarity to non-gestational parent
- Shared interests
- Race/ethnicity
- High sperm count (for sperm donors)
- Health history
- Mental health history
- Family genetic history
- IQ level
- Location
- Personal connection
- Cost efficacy
- Eye color
- Hair color
- _____
- _____

WHAT TRAITS ARE HEREDITARY, AND WHAT AREN'T?

It might surprise you, but there is actually much debate about this within the scientific community. Some studies and theories suggest that there are strong genetic determinants that shape our personalities, and others suggest that the way we are raised is more influential than where our genes come from.[1]

While we still don't know for sure where to land within the nature/nurture debate, some things are clear: Certain physical traits, like eye color, height, and melanin levels, are genetically inherited, although not always predictable—the way someone looks is formed through a complex formula based on the genes present in the sperm and egg cells that combine to form that particular person. It's possible that some personality traits, such as a person's timidity level or tendency to rebel against authority, have genetic components as well. However, various studies point out that a person's sense of connection, their ability to form deep relationships with others, is more strongly influenced by the ways they were raised than by where their genes came from. And one thing we know as queer folks is that love and strong parenting bonds transcend biological connection.

HOW TO MAKE YOUR DECISION

Awesome—you've identified important characteristics you want in your donor. Now circle your top five. After looking at your top five qualities, rank them in order of importance from one to five on the worksheet below. If you have a partner you're planning to build your family with, we recommend each of you do this exercise individually, as this can help foster important conversations between the two of you.[2]

My top five priorities in a donor are:

1.

2.

3.

4.

5.

Of these, my number one priority is:

When my child is ten, I will care that my donor…

Logistical ease is / is not more important to me than any of
the donor's characteristics. (circle your choice)

Still feeling overwhelmed? Ellie, a prospective solo parent by choice and friend of Marea's, shared with us this easy litmus test: *Imagine explaining to your future child why you chose this specific donor. Would you be able to explain your choice with confidence and with integrity?* If you can imagine having this conversation with your future child, you are on the right track.

What's the Difference Between Known Donors and Anonymous Donors?

Now that you've identified the qualities that are important to you in your donor, the next step is choosing *how* you would like to acquire sperm or eggs. There are two options for gathering the needed genetic material to create a pregnancy: known donors and anonymous donors. A known donor is someone from your life or community who agrees to provide sperm or eggs for the purpose of making a pregnancy. This person can be a friend, a family member of your partner, or a person you find on the internet. An anonymous donor is a person who donated their sperm or eggs to a cryobank to be purchased by individuals or families to aid in conception.

Why do people use known donors? Cost is a big factor. Known donors can appear to be free from the onset for people needing sperm, unlike purchasing vials of sperm from a cryobank. There is typically no essential cost to making a sperm donation, though some people do include monetary transactions in the donor contract (and we highly recommend you have a contract! More on that soon).

For people needing eggs, the cost of egg retrieval with a known donor is cheaper than purchasing eggs from an egg bank. If the person providing eggs also provides a uterus to carry the pregnancy—a process known as traditional surrogacy—the cost of conception may decrease dramatically. We will talk in depth about traditional surrogacy as well as other surrogacy options later in this chapter, but for now let's explore the ins and outs of using both known donors and anonymous donors to grow your family.

Considerations with Known Donors

Relationships

Known donors help us create unique family relationships and narratives, and for some individuals and families, having the donor participate in their child's life as a friend or family-like member is important for their family's story. Marea and her wife see their known donor about once a year, because they want their kids to have a relationship with him (but he isn't involved in any decisions or day-to-day stuff). When they invited their known donor to their wedding, they all took photos together, and they printed one out and put it up in their home. They wanted their kids to have a visual presence of their donor, to help them feel connected to where some of their ancestry and genetic material comes from.

We know some families that have the opportunity to use a known donor who is related to their partner, such as a cousin who donates sperm or a sister who donates eggs. This creates the added benefit of the family sharing a biological relationship, but it does require a very particular set of circumstances where all members are in agreement about the arrangement and committed to keeping everything drama-free.

> I don't remember ever considering using an anonymous donor. I wanted our donor to be someone we had a relationship with and who our kid could have a relationship with. So we ran through all our queer, cis male friends and pretty quickly knew we would ask Steve first. It just seemed practical. He was a close friend for a decade, and he and his partner were people we would want in our child's life long-term. Yes, we discussed qualities in Steve that we considered hereditary and liked, but that was not a large part of the decision. —Sauce Leon

The potential challenges of known donors include navigating these relationships in the long term. There can be issues if a donor has different expectations about their relationship with the child than the parents do. For example, they may want more or less involvement with the child than the parents are comfortable with, with the worst-case scenario being legal custody challenges after the birth. While initially planning a family is really exciting, heartwarming, and full of possibility, it's also important to think about what could happen if relationships change over time. Ask yourself: How would you navigate your family's situation if things got complicated?

Health Considerations
Knowing a potential donor's personal and family health history as well as any known genetic disorders may be an important factor in

deciding whether or not to create a child with them. Concerns about mental and physical illnesses that a potential donor or their family members carry can be a consideration for some individuals and families.

A genetic disease is an illness that is passed down in families through genes, which is something you or your potential donor may be a carrier for. Most genetic diseases require both genetic contributors to a pregnancy to be a carrier of the same condition, though some do not. Some people know they are a carrier for a particular illness that runs in their family, and others don't. Some of our clients opt to go through extensive genetic testing before conceiving to confirm whether or not they are carriers for any genetic disorders; others feel comfortable enough with what they know of their family health history and personal health to proceed without these tests. If you or a potential known donor have a family history of a genetic illness or know you may be a carrier, we recommend both parties have complete genetic testing prior to initiating donation.

Legal Considerations

We urge anyone using a known donor to create a written agreement or contract with their donor *before* initiating donation. The goal of that contract is to protect the parenting rights of the intended parents and to clarify expectations for all parties, including the current or future partner of a known donor. It also provides a framework for decision making, clarifying expectations, and the severing of the donor's parental rights, which can be important if there is a disagreement with the donor in the future. Donor agreements are viewed as legally binding contracts in some states, but not all. You can work with a family law attorney to draft a known donor agreement, or write one yourself. There are also some legal organizations that offer sliding-scale services for LGBTQ+ or solo parent families. We offer more information on legal considerations in chapter 9, and you can find a sample known donor contract on page 271.

For those creating a family with known donor eggs, rather than known donor sperm, the biological reality of the egg retrieval and donation process automatically creates some legal barriers. To donate eggs, medication, doctors, and freezing technology are all necessities, whereas donating sperm can potentially happen in someone's home without a healthcare provider.

According to Rebecca Levin Nayak, a family lawyer based in Philadelphia whom we consulted in the process of writing this book, fertility clinics performing egg retrievals for donation and IVF for surrogacy will often require the involvement of lawyers and legal agreements as part of the process. Sperm donation does not have this same legal barrier unless the insemination process involves a healthcare provider.

The only time this legal barrier is not created in the egg donation process is if a surrogate uses their own eggs to carry a pregnancy for another family, which is called traditional surrogacy. In these cases, families should meet with a lawyer prior to conception to draw up paperwork acknowledging this plan, but full parentage isn't established until after birth, when the traditional surrogate surrenders parenting rights to the intended parents through adoption. If you are using eggs from a known donor to create a family, you have more legal protections if the eggs are going into a different person's uterus.

The legal system has not caught up with the needs of LGBTQ+ and solo parent families, so the degree to which a known donor contract could hold up in court varies from state to state. Keep in mind that sample contracts found in this book or online may not reflect particular laws or language relevant to your state or country, so it's important to do research specific to where you live.

Regardless of whether you use a lawyer or do it yourself, any known donor agreement should address the following:

- What testing is required of the donor (see "Sexual Health, Genetics, and Lab Testing for Known Donors" below).
- How the donor will provide semen samples, and how many samples or how many egg retrievals they will undergo.
- The length of time you agree to try for a pregnancy.
- The names of the intended parents and that the donor does not have parental rights.
- The intended parents' expectations of the relationship with the donor in the event of pregnancy, miscarriage, and/or live birth.
- Statements from any partners of the donor that they agree to sperm or egg donation and to the donor relinquishing claims to parental rights.
- Financial obligations of the donor and intended parents.

Costs

It's customary for the family receiving egg or sperm donation to pay for expenses related to creating a pregnancy. When working with surrogates, intended parents are responsible for all legal, healthcare, and logistical fees for their surrogate as well. We will dive into all the expenses related to acquiring sperm, eggs, and uteruses in following sections.

HOW TO TALK TO YOUR KIDS ABOUT THEIR DONORS

It can be complex and sometimes very emotional to talk to our kids about how we made them or how they joined our family. Whether your donor is in your life and comes to every birthday party or you purchased gametes from a bank, it is important to be up front and honest with our children about how they came into this world.

I found out that my parents had used donor sperm to conceive my brother and me when my (sperm-donor-conceived) daughter was three, and it was an instant and drastic shift in perspective for me, despite being a queer parent who was super thoughtful going into the process of conceiving my child. There were *loads* of truths and identity elements that I hadn't ever thought of prior to actually experiencing it myself. It's a fairly huge topic and one that is filled with mixed emotions and lots of ongoing discussion, but also one that can often be missing in queer contexts where we've fought so hard to just be seen as valid parents within a larger heteronormative world. —Beth Gillis

The wider world often judges the validity of LGBTQ+ and solo parent families, which means speaking to our kids about their donors can be a long-term, ongoing discussion filled with mixed emotions. Still, it's important to be clear with our kids. On page 301, we offer a list of children's books particular to LGBTQ+ and solo parent families, some of which kid-splain donors in a lighthearted and accessible way.

Considerations with Anonymous Donors

An anonymous donor is a person who was paid to donate their sperm or eggs to a cryobank to be frozen for the purpose of helping other families create a pregnancy. Cryobanks take care of the work of pre-screening donors for health concerns by performing STI (sexually transmitted infection) and genetic screening, and also handle the legal concerns like severing donors' parental rights before sperm or eggs are available to purchase.

There are two types of donors at cryobanks: closed ID and open

ID. Closed ID donors are folks who do not want to be contacted by a child when they reach the age of eighteen. Open ID donors are open to being contacted by the children their eggs or sperm helped create once that child turns eighteen.

Open ID donors tend to cost slightly more; however, with the advent of genealogy testing, closed donors might become a thing of the past since children may be able to find their donor whether or not they want to be found. Some people argue that it is more ethical to choose open ID donors since many children become curious about their biological donors as they get older.[3]

Why do people use anonymous donors? Cryobanks offer prospective parents more control and relational safety in the family-building process. You do not have to navigate a personal relationship with your donor, and therefore there's little risk of potential conflicts. While eggs and sperm from a cryobank are expensive, the costs are up front and clear. The bank's health screening takes away risk of exposure to STIs. Many people like the simplicity of choosing a donor through the information provided by the sperm bank, versus the potentially messy and emotionally complicated choice of choosing a donor from the people they know.

We chose our donor because of how intellectual his profile made him seem. He had a job working in a scientific field and had high standardized test scores. We also were really charmed that he said he loved birds—we figured if you like birds, you're definitely a nice person. —Rachel

CONSIDERATIONS FOR SPERM DONATION

When you lack sperm and you see people with penises all around you, there can be a frustrating feeling that sperm is everywhere except where you need it most! Even though sperm may seem to be readily available yet just out of reach, there are a lot of factors that play into how different families choose their sperm donor.

This section is particularly for people using sperm donors to create a pregnancy in their or their partner's body. If you also need or intend to use an egg donor and surrogate, we'll address those considerations on page 41.

Known Donors—How Sperm Donation Works

For many people, a local known donor can seem like the most straightforward option for conception. This is what we've seen on TV for how people who were assigned female at birth get pregnant. What you don't see on TV is all the planning and decision making that goes into preparing for a pregnancy.

To conceive with a known donor, you can use fresh semen, or you can process and freeze the sperm at a cryobank to create a pregnancy later. Most people who use a known donor inseminate on their own, DIY-style, though some utilize a midwife or fertility clinic.

One of the reasons many people choose known donors is improved conception rates with fresh sperm. Fresh sperm can live for up to five days inside the body, whereas frozen sperm generally lives about twelve to twenty-four hours.[4] So, assuming your donor is local, there's a higher chance of conception with fresh sperm. We'll talk more about the details and review success rates with different conception methods in chapter 4. For now, let's go over the logistics of using a known donor.

Sexual Health, Genetics, and Lab Testing for Known Donors

Sexual health and safety are considerations when using a known donor. Using a known donor means exposing yourself to another person's sexual health practices. We recommend having a frank conversation with your potential donors about their current partners and sex life to determine if their sexual safety practices are okay with you. If your potential donor can't have an honest, clear conversation with you about their partners, dating, use of condoms, and STI risk, they might not be the best fit for sperm donation.

We were originally planning on having our known donor come over and donate fresh sperm when it was time to conceive. But in the time between agreeing that he would donate and when we were ready to conceive, two things happened: He got divorced and started dating, and the COVID-19 pandemic began. Because of the unknowns of how Covid was transmitted as well as our discomfort level around his sexual practices, we decided to bank his sperm at a cryobank and use frozen sperm to conceive. —Hannah R

We recommend that anyone using a known donor have them complete full STI testing, including HIV, hepatitis B, hepatitis C, syphilis, gonorrhea, and chlamydia, before proceeding with the insemination. Knowing your donor is not currently carrying any sexually transmitted infections protects the health of the person being inseminated and prevents fertility and pregnancy complications. When checking for STIs, other routine testing can include determining your donor's blood type, Rh factor, and CMV status, as well as genetic screening.

We have also found it to be worthwhile to ask donors to do a semen analysis before starting inseminations. While it may feel like an awkward conversation, a donor with a lower sperm count or low sperm motility will have fewer viable sperm to create a pregnancy. This could impact your ability to get pregnant and may change your decision to use that particular donor; if you still want to use that donor's sperm, having the information up front might direct you to opt for fertility treatments like IUI or IVF to create a pregnancy.

If the person who intends to use their eggs to create a pregnancy has a history of genetic diseases in their family or learns that they are a carrier for any genetic diseases, then checking to see if their donor is also a carrier for the genetic disease is an important part of their decision making. If both you and your donor are carriers for the same genetic disease, you may consider choosing a different donor, or talking to a genetic counselor about what it would be like to raise a child with a particular condition. Others choose to pursue advanced fertility treatments such as IVF that allow you to match unaffected eggs and sperm.

STI testing can typically be done without a provider's referral. If you have a sperm bank in your area, they may allow individuals to pay out of pocket to check their sperm count, but in most areas your donor will need a doctor's or a midwife's order to go to a lab for semen analysis. Genetic testing also must be ordered by a healthcare provider. At-home DNA tests like 23andMe are *not* genetic screenings and do not provide you with the clinical information you need to make family-planning decisions.

Depending on your donor's health insurance, these health screenings could be a few hundred dollars out of pocket that you should expect to pay for.

At least a few months before you plan to do your first insemination, get an extended genetic test. If you can, get the same genetic test that the sperm bank you are working with uses. You can call them to ask which company they use. If you use the same genetic testing company as the sperm bank, then you avoid a lot of hassle when you choose a donor and need to compare your test results with theirs (i.e., potential issues like being a carrier for a genetic disease that the donor wasn't tested for). —Ellie Lobovits

What If You Live Far Away from Your Donor?

Some people find their perfect sperm donor—but they live far away from them. If you live more than a few hours away from your donor, there are several logistical considerations to plan around that can add cost (and potentially stress) to the conception process.

If your donor does not live a reasonable distance to drive to last-minute, the options for working with them are (a) you or your donor traveling for inseminations; (b) banking and freezing the donor's sperm at a cryobank to then be shipped to you for inseminations with a midwife at home or at a fertility clinic; and (c) using a company that helps you ship fresh semen domestically overnight.

Banking and Freezing Known Donor Sperm

The process of banking your donor's sperm at a cryobank is called directed donor services. Sperm banks typically require your known donor to come in for a physical exam and extensive STI testing; after that they can give sperm deposits that can be processed and banked for later use. Sperm can be frozen washed or unwashed. Washed sperm has been treated with a chemical process to separate the semen from the sperm, which makes it safe for IUI (intrauterine insemination—in other words, the process of putting sperm cells directly into the uterus with a sterile catheter). Unwashed sperm has not gone through a chemical treatment, which makes it safe *only* for ICI (intracervical insemination, or the process of putting semen into the cervix) unless it's washed at the time of insemination. Washing costs a little bit more, but many folks choose to do this because IUI success rates with frozen sperm are higher than ICI success rates with frozen sperm.[5]

Per interpretation of FDA regulations, sperm banks require a six-month quarantine from the time sperm is deposited to when you can use it when you are not in a sexual relationship with your donor. Unfortunately, you still have to pay for sperm storage during this time. To complete the quarantine requirements, your donor must have full STI testing at the intake appointment, and then repeat the same STI tests six months after the last sperm deposit. This adds significant cost to the direct donor process and can be challenging for people trying to conceive now or yesterday. This FDA regulation results in one form of legal discrimination LGBTQ+ and other non-traditional families face.

The one workaround for people on a short timeline is that with the help of a provider, some sperm banks will allow clients to waive the six-month quarantine if the sperm samples are given the same week as the STI testing.[6] Ray learned about this FDA loophole from one of their clients a few years ago and, after calling around to the sperm banks near their known donor, found one bank willing to waive the quarantine with a letter from a healthcare provider. This loophole can be tricky to navigate within some fertility clinics but may work well for home or midwife inseminations.

If you are hoping to try to get pregnant six to twelve months from now, then you won't need to worry about these logistics, but you will need to factor in the cost of storage fees at your particular sperm bank.

The costs of direct donor deposits varies widely depending on the cryobank, geographic location, and whether you choose to freeze washed or unwashed sperm. As of this book's publication, the cost for directed donor services was between $3,700 and $5,500 for intake, base fees, testing, and up to one year of storage.

Shipping Fresh Sperm

There are companies that ship fresh sperm for home insemination. These companies typically put sperm in a chicken-egg-yolk buffer, which is the same technology that's used for animal husbandry. Does it work with human semen? Perhaps. People do get pregnant this way; however, there haven't yet been studies following how long human sperm lives through this mode of transport or rates of successful pregnancies conceived through home semen shipping. That said, a client of Ray's who tried this service allowed them to look at semen that had been shipped overnight under a microscope, and the sperm was very much alive!

Using a shipping kit to mail sperm overnight is a much more economical option than directed donor services with a bank, although again, we can't vouch for the success rates. At the time of this publication, each shipping kit costs between $130 and $200 before the cost of overnight shipping.

Anonymous Donors—How It Works

For those wanting more control and anonymity in their family-building process, purchasing sperm from a bank may make sense. There are two main types of sperm that can be purchased from a sperm bank: washed and unwashed sperm (return to page 33 for a refresher on the differences). It's helpful to know what insemination tool you plan to use *before* purchasing sperm from a bank, so that you can choose the correct type of sperm for you. We'll talk in depth about why people choose different insemination methods in chapter 4.

Sometimes when looking through a sperm bank website you will also see ART sperm samples. *ART* stands for "assisted reproductive technology," and the samples have a lower sperm count than washed or unwashed sperm samples. Unless you are utilizing advanced reproductive technologies plus in vitro fertilization to create your family, don't order this sperm.

Cost

The average cost of sperm varies widely. At the time of this writing, one vial ranges from $750 to $1,200. Unwashed sperm typically costs a bit less than washed. Shipping fees may be more than $200, and storage can run anywhere from $300 to $500 per year. Some banks allow customers to pick up sperm directly, which can save on shipping expenses. Cryobanks reevaluate their prices each year, and depending on the market and other factors, these prices can increase up to 10 percent annually.

How Much Sperm Should I Buy?

One of the quandaries that comes up when using sperm banks is how many vials to buy. A big question here is: Do you want multiple children? If you do, is it important to you that your children be genetically related? Frozen sperm can be stored for up to ten years, so if having genetically related children is a priority for you, buying more sperm may make sense. The average number of intrauterine inseminations it takes to achieve a pregnancy for people under thirty-five with no fertility issues is four. The numbers get a little trickier to predict, statistically, for people over thirty-five. But the most common recommendation is that if you want one child, purchase four sperm vials, and if you want two children, purchase eight.

That said, buying so many vials at once isn't financially feasible for many people. To avoid storage fees, we've had clients who purchase one sperm vial at a time. If you choose to go this route, you may have to switch from donor to donor if a particular donor sample runs out, or to purchase sperm earlier than planned if your perfect donor is running low. We know that these decisions can be stressful. No matter what you decide, remember that your main goal is to make a baby, and your donor is just one of the steps in getting you there.

ARE SOME SPERM BANKS BETTER THAN OTHERS?

It's hard to say. Aside from FDA rules on infectious disease testing, the sperm bank industry in the United States is largely unregulated and, except for the Sperm Bank of California in Berkeley, all for-profit. One of the key things to look for when choosing a sperm bank is how many donor-conceived children they allow per donor. The American Society for Reproductive Medicine recommends no more than twenty-five births per donor.[7]

How to Choose an Anonymous Sperm Donor

Looking through a sperm bank website can be a very surreal experience. The idea of picking your child's genes from a pool of strangers is overwhelming for some and pretty simple for others. A client of Marea's once described it as online dating, but for genetic material.

> Choosing a sperm donor after years of online dating took a bit of a mind shift. The process of looking through profiles was so similar but I had to continuously remind myself that the nineteen-year-old in the picture wasn't too young for me—I was looking for sperm, not a partner.
> —Meredith Nutting

Before you even start to look for a donor, the most important thing is to choose your three biggest priorities. (Hint: Look at your three top-ranked qualities from the exercise on page 21.) Everyone's top three will be different, but often those priorities include a similar ethnic background as the non-gestational parent (if applicable) as well as similar physical features, level of education, interests, or personality traits. If you're feeling overwhelmed by picking a donor from a cryobank's website, you are not alone! Many prospective parents feel daunted by this task.

When going about this process of finding a donor from a bank, we recommend trying not to get overly analytical about your choice. As we mentioned on page 20, some traits are hereditary (like eye color) and others are more nurture-based (like someone's ability to connect with others).[8]

When you're ready to dive into the cryobank websites, stick to your top three priorities. Make a small collection of donor options and see which one resonates with you the most. Sperm banks offer lots of extra features for picking donors for an additional fee. These extras can include more pictures, voice recordings, interviews, and more. For some people, details like listening to a donor's voice really matter, but for others, these features can be part of a rabbit hole that makes it even more difficult to decide. Remember: Decision fatigue is real! We recommend sticking with a small group of viable options and making the simplest choices whenever possible.

> Picking out sperm was creepy for me. We made the mistake of listening to one of the recorded donor profile interviews. Hearing the voice of some twenty-two-year-old frat boy trying to pretend like his motivation was to help people build families was unsettling to me. I was obsessed with finding a donor profile that was up front about their intentions. Finally, we settled on a short list that I felt was authentic. —Jennifer Soady

Sometimes, if you call a sperm bank and say that you're going to purchase sperm that day, they will give you access to additional features at no added cost. Another interesting fact about sperm banks is that they have sales! If you have some time before you want to begin inseminations, get on a few sperm banks' listservs, save your top-choice donors, and then wait for a sale to purchase the sperm vials.

A Note About Sperm Donors and Race

There are significant racial disparities in available donor sperm. The low rates of donor sperm of color are well documented, with shortages in Black, Asian, Middle Eastern, and Filipino donors, among others. In a 2020 review of the California cryobank sperm donor registry by Angela Hatem, of the 433 total donors, 260 were Caucasian, and 15 were African American.[9]

There are a number of reasons for this. Hatem notes that sperm banks are typically located in mostly white areas and use the same marketing strategies to recruit Black donors and other donors of color that they use to recruit white donors. There is also a long history of US medical institutions experimenting on Black people's bodies, which leaves many Black communities feeling mistrustful of modern Western medical institutions. The racial makeup of clinic staff may also make Black and brown donors feel unwelcome and not interested in returning.[10]

For many clients of color, finding a sperm donor with the same ancestry or ethnic background as themselves or their partner is an extra hurdle in addition to all the emotional and financial costs of choosing a donor. As it does with everything, racism plays a role in families' conception options.

We are a queer, genderqueer, and multiracial family. I (Mama, they/she) am a Black Chinese queer and genderqueer settler, and I birthed our eight-month-old. My partner and co-parent (Abba, they/them) is a white queer and trans settler. We chose our sperm donor from a sperm bank.

We knew we were going to raise a Black queer kid. When I say queer, I mean politically queer, as our kid was going to be raised with values that center and embrace agency, sovereignty, and creative expansiveness as it pertains to lived experiences and embodiments of gender and sexuality. And when I say—and capitalize—Black here, I mean racially and politically Black, as our kid was going to be raised in a household where *Black* means liberation and future; an end to policing, borders, and carceral construction; and decolonial imagination.

So when we looked at the sperm bank and saw that out of the seven Black donors three of them worked for law enforcement, we knew what our first criteria was: *No cops.* This is not because we harbor false notions that being a cop is genetically predispositioned but rather because when our Black queer kid grows up going to direct actions, learning from artist/activist elders, and processing their lived experience through the lenses and lessons of Black feminism, Abolitionists, and Land and Water Defenders, we wanted them to also know and feel that the thought and values that went into their coming into being were emblematic of the practices of worlding that we would spend our lives enacting alongside them. —Mila Mendez

Purchasing sperm from a sperm bank is both an odd and a straightforward process. Uniquely, you get to choose your child's DNA, and the bank takes care of the legal considerations of sperm donation and severing parenting rights of the donor, making the legal formation of your family simpler.

Frozen sperm, however, is expensive. The conception rates with frozen sperm are lower than with fresh sperm, which can leave you with the additional cost of using a midwife or reproductive endocrinologist to assist with insemination procedures to improve conception rates. Lack of Black, Latino, Native American, Middle Eastern, and Asian donors means family-building options through anonymous donation are limited or out of reach for many. And while many parents love the simplicity and anonymity, it's important to consider that donor-conceived children's needs may possibly differ from those of their parents. Studies indicate that often, donor-conceived kids want some level of connection to their donor later in life.[11] For this reason, when choosing sperm from a bank, we recommend considering open ID donors who consent to potentially meeting the child when they are eighteen.

CONSIDERATIONS FOR EGG DONORS, UTERUSES, AND SURROGACY

Egg donors and surrogacy offer one possible path to parenthood for gay men, trans women, and people who don't have a uterus in their relationship and want genetically related children. Other folks may consider exploring egg donors and surrogacy as well, even if they have a uterus, such as people who have certain fertility issues that make pregnancy difficult or life threatening, or professional athletes who want to have children without sacrificing their careers.

Families in need of eggs and a uterus to have genetically related children have a two-step process of choosing an egg donor as well as somebody willing to gestate their child. While the process of conceiving when using someone else's eggs and uterus is often more medicalized and expensive, IVF success with surrogacy and donor eggs is extremely high—resulting in live births up to 80 percent of the time after one cycle.[12]

As we walk you through the costs and logistics of building a family with egg donation and surrogacy, we want to warn that we are going to be talking about costs that may feel disheartening and out of reach. We'll discuss grants and insurance coverage later in this chapter, as well as in the appendix on page 284, but it feels important to name that financial inaccessibility and lack of insurance coverage is a form of discrimination LGBTQ+ people and solo parents face in growing our families.

Some people reading this section may lack just eggs or a uterus in their relationship, not both. Since the need for one typically means a need for the other, we'll be talking about the two processes in tandem, but egg donation, IVF, and surrogacy can be done independently.

Eggs can come from a cryobank or from a family member, friend, partner, or person on the internet. The process of harvesting eggs involves the donor taking hormones to increase the total number of eggs produced per reproductive cycle; once the eggs have reached a certain level of maturity, the donor is placed under anesthesia and the eggs are retrieved. Following collection, donor eggs can be stored in an egg bank or fertilized with sperm to create an embryo to implant into another person's uterus or stored for future use. Donor eggs are used in about 12 percent of all IVF cycles in the United States annually with high success rates, which makes them an effective tool for creating a pregnancy.[13]

I always knew I wanted to be a father. I also knew that it would be difficult and expensive as a gay man, but this was something I'd hoped and planned for for years. I was just waiting for a partner, and gave myself the deadline of forty to start the process. As I was still single the day after my fortieth birthday, I threw myself into researching surrogacy and egg donation. It took several weeks—countless hours really—to research my road map ahead. There was no single platform that provided all the information I needed around where to start the surrogacy process, which included finding a surrogacy agency, an egg donor, and a fertility clinic. I had to create extensive spreadsheets just to keep track of all the different agencies and egg donors I was considering and to be able to compare my options. Despite all my best planning, there were still a lot of surprises and confusion along the way.

One of the best parts of my story is that a few months after meeting my gestational carrier, I met my husband, Dr. Michael Gowen, and we've been parenting together ever since. We were married two years later and now have a sister for Ariel: Yael, also born via surrogacy and egg donation. —Eran Amir, founder of GoStork

Known Versus Anonymous Egg Donors

We discussed some of the pros and cons of known donors versus anonymous donors regarding navigating relationships and unique family narratives earlier in this chapter. One of the primary differences in creating families with donor eggs versus donor sperm is that there are two paths with distinctly different legal implications. If a known donor does not want to carry a pregnancy with their eggs for another family, they can donate their eggs. However, if a known donor carries a pregnancy for another family using their own eggs, they are considered a legal parent until they surrender their parenting rights after birth. While called "traditional" surrogacy, the risk tolerance and trust required make this method of surrogacy less common.

When growing your family through surrogacy, some families

find their surrogate before choosing an egg donor, while others choose the egg donor and create frozen embryos before choosing the person who will carry the baby for them. Since frozen embryos last for at least ten years, you do have the option to freeze them and save them for the future.[14] It is customary for intended parents to cover the costs of egg retrieval when using a known donor, as well as all costs of family building through surrogacy.

Egg cryobanks are similar to sperm cryobanks (in fact, many cryobanks carry both sperm and eggs) in that you create a login and search donor profiles, having access to information about the donor's life, health, education, and physical features. You have the option to purchase closed ID or open ID donors, which refers to whether future children would have the ability to contact their donor at age eighteen. When choosing an egg donor, find your top three priorities and try not to get bogged down in the rest—the worksheet offered at the beginning of this chapter is meant to support you in this process.

My husband has a younger sister, and when we were talking about growing our family, we thought: How cool would it be if we could use her eggs and my sperm so that our children could be biologically related to us both? When we first asked her, she said no...not because she didn't want to be a donor, but because she was phobic of needles and the whole IVF process was intimidating to her. So we let the idea go. But then, six months later, my mom suggested that we ask again, but offer her tons of support around the whole process. This time, she agreed. We had a close family friend help with the injections and then we got to create tons of embryos that were products of both my husband and me. —Neill Sullivan

EGG DONORS AND RACE

The same lack of diversity in donors exists in egg banks as in sperm banks, although the shortage of African American donors is not as severe. In her research, Angela Hatem found that Egg Donor America, one of America's leading egg donation agencies, had four hundred Caucasian donors available, the category labeled "African" yielded sixteen possible donors, and "African American" turned up one hundred.[15] Availability of egg donors of color is very much location-dependent. There are shortages of Afro-Caribbean, Indian, Asian, and Jewish egg donors.[16]

Buying Eggs

Once you've selected your donor, the next question is: How many eggs do you need? The recommendation from most fertility clinics is six to eight. The reason for this is that not all eggs fertilized during IVF will create an embryo, and not all embryos will grow enough to be implanted into the uterus. Typically 80 percent of eggs thawed will survive being fertilized, and 30 to 50 percent of fertilized eggs will grow into a blastocyst.

The combo of egg donation, IVF, and surrogacy does have significantly high success rates, sometimes achieving a clinical pregnancy rate of 86 percent and live birth rate of 80 percent after one cycle, compared with an average birth rate of 46.2 percent using donor eggs for IVF in the general population.[17] At the time of this book's publication, a batch of five to seven donor eggs costs anywhere from $17,000 to $25,000,[18] which may or may not include shipping to the fertility clinic or storage.

In comparison, when a friend or family member donates their

eggs, an egg retrieval/freezing cycle typically costs about $8,000 and egg or embryo storage costs around $500 per year. It's slightly better to freeze embryos than eggs, because embryos have a better chance of survival. There is a risk in using a known donor that an egg retrieval cycle will not be successful, or that there will not be enough viable eggs to create a successful embryo.

There are several factors that play into what makes some retrieval cycles more successful than others. Age of the egg donor is one of the primary factors, with egg donors under thirty having the highest likelihood of creating successful embryos. Also, be aware that sometimes FDA rules around egg donation and infectious disease screening can put some stress on the IVF timeline because the clinic can require a lot of appointments and testing for the egg donor around the time of egg retrieval.

Surrogates

A surrogate is a person with a uterus who uses their body to grow a pregnancy for another family, known as the intended parents. As we've discussed, there are two kinds of surrogacy: traditional surrogacy, where the person whose uterus you're going to use is also using their own eggs; and gestational surrogacy or gestational carrier, where the person who will carry the pregnancy for another family does not share genetic material with the fetus, and the intended parents use donor eggs and IVF to conceive.

As midwives we have both seen unique wonderful bonds formed between gestational carriers and intended parents, particularly when the power relationship is equal and both parties are part of a supportive experience.

The main reason most surrogates use donor eggs instead of their own eggs is that it creates legal separation between the gestational surrogate and the intended parents. If the surrogate is using their own eggs, legally, the child is considered theirs and, in those circumstances, the surrogate must be willing to have their parental rights severed from the child following the birth. If the egg that created the pregnancy is not from the surrogate's body, there are more legal protections for the intended parents. In most states, the intended parents can get a "pre-birth order" certifying them as parents through the birth certificate.

Traditional surrogacy can appeal to some families because it can remove the cost of egg retrieval and IVF. These relationships require a lot of trust and mutual understanding, as well as many contracts and legal counseling before, during, and after pregnancy, so that the intended parents may gain full parental rights.

Working with a Surrogate

Surrogacy is an incredibly intimate relationship, because it requires immense trust for one person to carry a pregnancy for another family.

There are two pathways to finding a surrogate to carry a pregnancy for your family. The first is to independently find a gestational carrier/ gestational surrogate, either from a person in your own community or by recruiting a surrogate independently through ads, fertility clinics, Facebook groups, or networking.[19] Sometimes queer people with uteruses, knowing the difficulty queer and trans people with penises face in family building, will be surrogates for our community.

When you're pursuing surrogacy independently of an agency, once you find a surrogate, the next step is finding a family lawyer specializing in surrogacy to draw up contracts. With both traditional surrogacy and gestational carriers, the legal agreements should be in place *before* starting the conception process. These agreements typically cover parental rights, medical decision-making, place of delivery, future contact, health insurance, payment of medical bills, liability with medical insurance and complications, compensation, lost wages, legal fees, childcare, housekeeping, maternity clothes, life insurance, participation of all parties in doctor visits, and information about medical history. There may be different considerations for financial support with traditional surrogacy than with gestational carriers. Be sure to work with a family lawyer who is familiar with the laws of your state, and who has experience with surrogacy in LGBTQ+ or solo families. (More information about legal considerations is available in chapter 9.)

The second pathway to family building with surrogacy is working with an agency that matches intended parents with a gestational surrogate. Here, intended parents are pre-screened before establishing a profile and meeting potential gestational surrogates. Working with a surrogacy agency costs significantly more than independent surrogacy, but agencies do provide a streamlined system for all legal, logistical, and physical concerns throughout the process.[20]

Surrogacy agencies bill themselves as one-stop shops, but it's important to get clarity on exactly what services are covered within their fees, what's not covered, and how they work with surrogates. Ask for an itemized list, and ask questions including:

- What's included in the agency's fee? When are fees due? What type of payment schedule or payment plans are available?
- What legal services are included in the fee? Will I need to hire an outside lawyer for anything else—and if so do you have connections to lawyers you work with and an estimate of the cost?
- How do you screen gestational carriers? What does the matching process look like? How are gestational surrogates paid? What percentage of matches result in successful live births? What support does the agency provide if a conflict develops between the gestational carriers and the intended parents?
- How are insurance and medical care for gestational carriers managed? Are those costs included, and if not, how much are they? Are any fertility clinic costs included?

Choosing a surrogacy agency is a big decision, and it may make sense to interview more than one agency before deciding who to work with. You can also ask agencies for references from former clients—both intended parents and surrogates, and fertility clinics they work with frequently. Pay special attention to the experience you have with the agency. For example, is the agency easy to navigate and responsive? Does it appear that gestational carriers are well treated? Write pro and con lists and price out options, but also listen to your instincts about what feels most right. Some of the costs presented by a surrogacy agency may be negotiable—make sure to check with the agency as well as the IVF clinic.

A NOTE ABOUT INTERNATIONAL SURROGACY

Most surrogacy occurring in the world does not have a shared power relationship between parties. Worldwide, the international surrogacy industry primarily consists of poor women of color from the Global South carrying babies for wealthy, primarily white families. Because of the exploitation of low-income women's bodies and the extreme power inequity in these relationships, most European countries have banned surrogacy, as have some states within the US. We urge you to consider the power balance when working with a surrogate, and whether or not the surrogate has full bodily autonomy. We wish for a world where all LGBTQ+ and solo folks can become parents in the ways they want to *and* that everyone involved has full agency and respect in the process.

Choosing a Surrogate

When you're meeting with potential surrogates for your family, whether through an agency or in your community, it's crucial to discuss all the potential points of conflict that may arise during conception, pregnancy, and birth. Details to consider include prenatal care and birth desires, feelings about genetic screening and pregnancy termination, diet and health practices, environmental exposures, travel, pumping breast milk, and if a surrogate is open to carrying future children for that family. While perfect alignment may be unattainable, having these uncomfortable conversations up front can help determine if everyone is a good match and prevent potential stress and conflict.

> "Mom Wanted." We wondered what to do—hang up a neon sign? Place an ad? Three polyamorous would-be dads need a biologic mom and surrogate? The idea of shopping for moms through an agency seemed palatable but not ideal. In the end we found our moms by offer, not by request. Two moms offered to donate embryos they couldn't use—that's what started us off. Two wonderful women heard my partner talking about our plans and offered to be an altruistic surrogate and an engaged, kind of "outside mom." We even got an unexpected breast milk donation (a year's worth!) from a nurse at my daughter's hospital! We three dads ended up owing everything to the generosity of five women.
> —Ian Jenkins, author of *Three Dads and a Baby*

Surrogacy Costs

So how much does surrogacy cost? If you're going through a US-based agency, fees can range from $90,000 to $150,000, including initial screenings and matching ($4,000 to $15,000), payment to the gestational carrier ($35,000 to $50,000), expenses related to carrying a pregnancy including medical coverage, lost work, and life insurance

($10,000 to $30,000), additional costs for twins and cesarean birth ($3,000 to $15,000), legal fees ($4,000 to $15,000), and agency fees (varies around $20,000 to $30,000, typically 15 to 25 percent of the total cost).[21] The cost may or may not include IVF and egg donor expenses.

> We used a surrogate coordinator through an agency who connects prospective parents with surrogates to find both of our surrogates. It's definitely more expensive to use an agency, and some of the fees do feel onerous, so I wouldn't honestly give a raving review because I do feel like some of the clinics have excessive fees. But with respect to the surrogates, I felt really good about paying them, paying them extra, and sending them food. That all felt great. They didn't deserve any less for all the physical and emotional labor they were doing to help us grow our family. —Neill Sullivan

Costs for surrogacy independent of an agency can include legal fees ($8,000 to $13,000[22]), the cost of fertility procedures and egg donor fees, and prearranged payment to your gestational carrier to cover anything from organic food to housecleaning, lost work, and compensation for surrogacy services.

Building families through egg donation and surrogacy is a multi-step process involving lawyers, fertility clinics, and community. The expenses of donor eggs, IVF, and surrogacy are significant, but sometimes minimized through using a known donor or community member as a surrogate. Traditional surrogacy, which can be an affordable path for family building when you lack a uterus and eggs, is also legally complex. Regardless of which path you pursue, it is an incredibly intimate experience to entrust another person to grow your baby.

We've covered a lot of information on how to acquire eggs, sperm, and a uterus. While it can be overwhelming to consider, we hope that you can also connect to the sweetness of beginning to grow your family. Once you choose a donor, you are that much closer to creating the person whose diapers you will change a million times. While choosing a donor may feel intense with all the decisions you need to make, parenting itself also bombards you with tons of necessary decisions, sometimes all at once. So maybe we just consider this phase practice?

Now that we know about our options for finding sperm, eggs, and a uterus, we're going to talk about how to put everything together.

CHAPTER 3

Timing Is Everything: How to Figure Out Your Fertility

As LGBTQ+ and solo people who want to create children within our own bodies without abundant access to sperm, timing inseminations well can really make or break our ability to get pregnant. In this chapter we'll walk you through what you need to understand your fertility and figure out when to inseminate to optimize the chances of getting pregnant. We'll go over the menstrual cycle (a little refresher from sixth-grade sex ed), as well as all the different ways that you can track your ovulation. We will also talk about what you can do (and not do) to support your fertility. In the next chapter, we go into depth about the different insemination options.

This chapter is all about understanding fertility as an important part of your baby-making journey. The bulk of this chapter is oriented toward people with uteruses who are planning to get pregnant. If that's not you, you can jump to page 90, where you'll find information about sperm health, and a section on optimizing fertility that contains information for people with eggs or sperm. If you're currently on T and considering going off to try to get pregnant or use your eggs in another person's body, consider jumping to chapter 5 to learn about trans fertility needs, and then come back to this chapter.

First Things First: What Is Fertility?

The term *fertility* refers to someone's potential to create offspring, and it encompasses oh so many things. We can think of fertility very broadly as a measure of one's potential to contribute healthy gametes to create and (if relevant) carry a pregnancy. For people with uteruses, fertility relates to the menstrual cycle and how our bodies produce different hormones that trigger ovulation at the midway point of our cycles. Fertility can also refer to the amount of sperm in someone's ejaculate as well as their shape and ability to travel to reach an egg.

For people with uteruses, understanding fertility is intrinsically connected to understanding the menstrual cycle. When we pay attention to and track all the symptoms occurring during the cycle, we can then identify our fertile (ovulatory) windows. If you are someone with a uterus who does not currently have a menstrual cycle and want to create a pregnancy in your own body, check out pages 59 and 79 for more information about learning about your fertility and health.

Ray, who has been co-teaching a queer and solo parent conception class called Beyond the Baster since 2018, sees that many people struggle to relate what is happening during the menstrual cycle to their conception process (even when using period-tracking apps). This chapter will help you understand what is happening inside your uterus, ovaries, and fallopian tubes throughout your menstrual cycle and how you can apply this knowledge to timing inseminations.

What's Actually Going on Inside the Uterus? Sex Ed 2.0

Your uterus, an organ about the size of your fist, lives right behind your pubic bone. If you push your fingers down firmly right above your pubic bone, you may be able to feel the very top of your uterus, which we call the fundus. When pushing down, you may feel a little pressure at the top of your vagina or front hole (or whatever other word you like to use to refer to that part of your body). That pressure is coming from your cervix, which looks like a turtleneck at the base of the uterus (check out the image on page 55 for a visual).

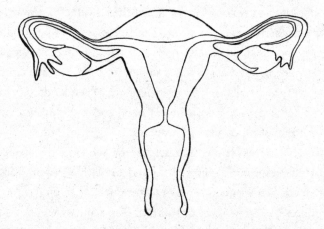

The cervix has many functions, from protecting your uterus from bacteria to holding babies inside it. By squatting and reaching inside the vagina / front hole with two fingers, most people will be able to feel their cervix. It's a small donut-shaped organ that has about the same consistency as your nose. Your cervix offers clues about your fertility throughout your cycle, which we will talk more about later.

Reaching out from both sides of your uterus are two fallopian tubes that each connect to an ovary. If you lie on your back and gently palpate yourself right above each groin, you may be able to feel your ovaries (no worries if you can't; Ray can't feel theirs). Each is about the size of a small almond. Your ovaries contain hundreds of thousands of eggs, one of which (or sometimes two) matures each cycle and is then released into its corresponding fallopian tube, where it awaits a potential sperm cell. People assigned female at birth are born with about one million eggs, but only a few hundred mature during the reproductive years.[1]

Let's Talk About Menstruation

In our culture, there is a lot of baggage around menstruation, and understandably so, given the pervasiveness of homophobia, transphobia, and sexism in this world that is directed toward people who menstruate. From a young age, people who menstruate are taught to be ashamed of their bodies. We internalize messages that this very normal bodily process is somehow gross. Menstruation can also be very gendered, and if our experience of gender doesn't match with society's expectations of what our gender should be, societal shame can be compounded by dysphoria.

Our goal in this chapter is to help people who menstruate deepen their understanding of their cycle and ovulation, leaving out the problematic gender stereotypes or assumptions that often come with this education. We will use anatomical terms and queer community language for reproductive body parts. There's nothing gross, wrong, or inherently feminine about uterine bleeding.

Four Phases in Every Cycle

Menstruation occurs in cycles, and these cycles are based on hormonal fluctuations. Most people who bleed experience a cycle that occurs more or less monthly. The average cycle is twenty-eight days long, though it's common for people to have cycles that range between twenty-one and thirty-six days (having a cycle that is more frequent than twenty days or longer than thirty-seven may indicate a health issue that could also cause challenges to getting pregnant—we'll talk more about that later in this chapter).

There are four main phases during each menstrual cycle: the menses phase, the follicular phase, the ovulatory phase, and the luteal phase. Or in other terms: bleeding, egg-maturation, egg-release, and body-preparing-for-possible-pregnancy. Identifying each of these phases is the first step toward understanding when you are the most fertile.

The first phase, menses, is when the uterus releases its uterine lining and lasts somewhere between two and seven days. Some people who bleed often think of their period as the end of the cycle, but when you're tracking fertility, the first day of bleeding is actually considered the *first* day of the cycle. While this may feel counterintuitive at first, it will make more sense when we get to determining ovulation.

The second phase of the cycle is the follicular phase, where the body, specifically the ovaries, prepares for ovulation. During this phase, your ovary releases the hormone estrogen, which causes the uterine lining to grow and thicken, and the brain releases follicle stimulating hormone, or FSH, which matures the egg within the ovaries. The follicular phase generally begins once people stop bleeding, around day five, and continues until ovulation.

After the egg matures, we enter the ovulatory phase, during which the ovary releases the matured egg. This third phase is the most crucial when it comes to fertility tracking. It's governed by the luteinizing hormone (LH), which is the hormone released by the brain that signals to the ovaries that it is time to release the egg into the fallopian tubes. LH typically spikes about twenty-four to thirty-six hours before your body releases the matured egg, but there can be a wide variation in this timing that depends on a variety of factors. Once an egg is released, it is viable for twelve to twenty-four hours. This is the window when an egg can be fertilized.

WHAT IS MITTELSCHMERZ?

Mittelschmerz is a German word for "middle pain," and it refers to the pain or sensation that some people experience within their ovaries during ovulation. Not everyone experiences mittelschmerz, but if you do, this can offer a great clue into when your ovary releases its egg.

After ovulation, the fourth and final phase is called the luteal phase. During the luteal phase, the ovaries produce the hormones progesterone and estrogen to prepare the uterus for a pregnancy to implant. If, during ovulation, sperm and egg meet and fertilize in the fallopian tube, and if this little zygote implants itself inside the uterine walls about five or six days later, the body continues producing

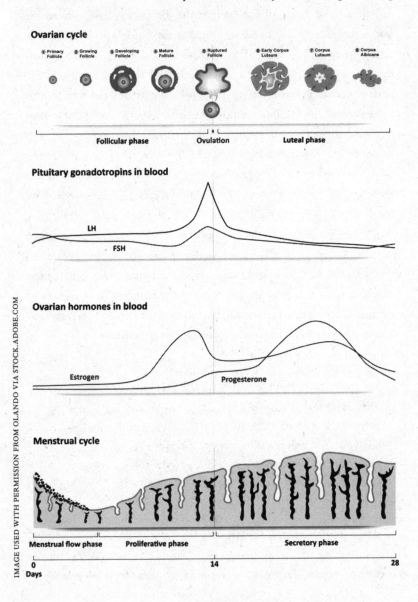

more estrogen and progesterone to support the embryo to continue growing. If pregnancy doesn't occur during this cycle, estrogen and progesterone levels rise for about twelve days then drop, causing menstruation. Then we go back to square one.

That's All Cool, but How Do I Know When I'm Ovulating?

Humans generally ovulate fourteen days *before* they get their period. So that means, if your cycle lasts for twenty-six days, you will most likely ovulate around day twelve; if your cycle is thirty-two days long, you'll probably ovulate around day eighteen. That said, people aren't robots! It's common for our cycles to change slightly—one month, we have a thirty-day cycle, the next a thirty-two-day cycle, and so on.

LET'S DO MATH!

Count how many days your last cycle was, and subtract fourteen from that number. The answer to this math problem is the day that you ovulated during your last cycle.

Since we can't time inseminations backward from our last period, that's where fertility tracking—and not just period tracking with apps—comes in. Learning how to track your body's fertile signs will help you anticipate when you ovulate, and as we said at the beginning: The more accurately you know when you're ovulating, the better you can time your inseminations and make a baby.

What If I Don't Have a Regular Cycle?

Again, some fluctuation is normal and expected. Some people, however, have irregular cycles, meaning that there is more than a four-day variation in length between one cycle and the next. For example, one cycle may be twenty-six days long, the next thirty-one days, and the next twenty-four days. With irregular cycles, it can be challenging to track your fertility and determine ideal insemination timing. If you have cycles that are shorter than twenty days or longer than thirty-seven, this can be an indication of *anovulation*—cycles where an egg is not released.

If you're interested in using your eggs and uterus to create a baby and don't have regular cycles, there are some nutrition, lifestyle, and holistic interventions that can support ovulation health and cycle regularity. We talk in depth about lifestyle, nutrition, and supplements that support fertility toward the end of this chapter on page 82.

If you have very long, short, or irregular cycles, we recommend having a pre-conception checkup with a midwife or doctor to screen for and treat the medical conditions that could be affecting your cycle's regularity. We talk about conditions that can cause anovulatory cycles on page 79, and how to find the right provider for you on page 127.

If, after making these changes and consulting with a provider, your cycle remains irregular, you may be prescribed medication that induces ovulation (more information on this in chapter 4). Even if you're on medication, as long as you're ovulating, it's possible to track your fertility with the methods we outline below.

Fertility Tracking

We'll level with you: Some people like fertility tracking, and others don't. Ray deeply dislikes cycle tracking, which they find ironic because they teach other people how to do it all the time. Still, for people with uteruses, fertility tracking is an essential tool in family creation. The alternatives to tracking your own fertile signs—visits to fertility clinic, ultrasounds, blood work, and medication—are expensive, and many people don't have insurance that will cover these costs.

They also don't necessarily improve conception rates for people with no confirmed fertility issues. So learning to track your fertility really is worth it, even if it feels annoying and overwhelming at times.

If you're a person with a uterus and a regular cycle, your body's main fertility signs are cervical position and openness, cervical fluid, basal body temperature, and levels of luteinizing hormone. Together, these four indicators can help you develop an understanding of your ovulation window and will help increase your chances of conception. Let's look at each one, and how to track it, in more detail. We recommend, if possible, spending a few months getting familiar with all your fertile signs *before* you start trying to conceive, so that you can optimize your chances of conception.

Cervical Position and Openness

As midwives, we are huge fans of the cervix. Cervixes do so many things! They move in different directions during the cycle, aligning with the vagina / front hole during menstruation and ovulation, then moving backward toward the tailbone at other times. They close firmly to keep babies inside during pregnancy and open to get babies out. They change color and texture, and they visibly open during ovulation to invite sperm inside the uterus. The website www .beautifulcervix.com shows tons of photos of cervixes throughout the menstrual cycle and will help you visualize this amazing organ and all the changes it goes through.

Checking your cervix's position and openness, whether feeling it with your fingers or viewing it with a speculum (or both!), gives you a very useful window into your fertility. Changes in your cervical position and openness may offer key information that will help you determine your ovulation and give you the most accurate sense of when to inseminate. Checking the cervix helps many feel more connected to their body and all the amazing things it does throughout the cycle. However, if you're somebody who just isn't comfortable feeling or looking at your cervix, that's okay! We go over other tools for tracking fertility later in this chapter, which may be more up your alley—feel free to skip ahead.

Feeling Your Cervix

During your period, the cervix opens so that the uterus can release its lining. Then, during the follicular phase, the cervix is closed, firm, and pointed toward your tailbone. During this phase, the consistency of the cervix feels like that of your nose. As ovulation approaches, the cervix starts to soften, open, and align with the vagina. You can imagine it as a tunnel, awaiting the potential of sperm. Now it begins to feel softer and squishier, more like your lips. The day of ovulation, the cervix is the most high, soft, and open that it will be throughout the entire cycle. This is the day to inseminate!

The day after ovulation, the cervix begins to close again, and it becomes firmer, gets lower in the body, and starts moving back toward the pubic bone. The cervical os (the opening of the cervix)

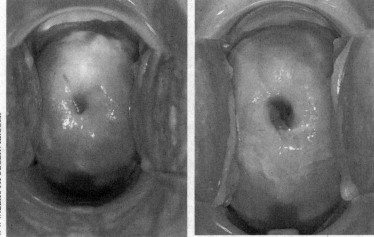

Photo of cervix on day 4 of cycle (not ovulating); photo of cervix on day 15 of cycle (ovulating)

closes completely within a day or two of ovulation and remains closed and firm for the remainder of the cycle.

You can feel your cervix yourself, or you can do this with a partner. Doing it yourself entails getting into a position that allows you to feel your cervix (squatting or sitting on a toilet seat is great) and using your index and middle fingers on your dominant hand to reach inside the vagina / front hole to touch the cervix. If you're doing this with a partner, lying on your back in a comfortable position works for most people. When tracking for fertility timing, we recommend checking your cervix once in the morning and once in the evening starting three or four days before you expect to ovulate.

A few pro tips for feeling your cervix:

- Wash your hands!
- Use lube (we recommend coconut oil or an organic water-based lubricant).
- Squat, or lift up one leg—any position that helps bring your hand within closer reach of the bottom half of your body works.
- Your cervix is about as firm as your nose, and it is shaped like a donut. If you or your partner can't feel it immediately when inside, try moving your fingers back and down slightly, closer to your sacrum.
- If you are feeling your partner's cervix, always make sure to have open, clear communication, and let them know what you are doing before you do it.

During the preparation phase before our first insemination attempt, the labor of queer family making felt powerful and intentional. I learned so much about the cycles of my body; after a few weeks, I was adept at finding my own cervix and got to share this knowledge with my wife. We celebrated the miraculous possibilities of the cervix and marveled at the sight, knowing that for people who want to and are able to give birth vaginally, the baby's head passes through that (currently) tiny cervix. As I began to understand the clues and cues of my reproductive cycle, I felt hopeful and a closeness with my own body. —Nikiko Masumoto

Visualizing Your Cervix

You can also look at your cervix with a speculum. This is Marea's favorite method for tracking ovulation because, to her, it offers the most concrete information for insemination timing. When the cervix is the most open, it's the perfect time to put sperm inside the uterus.

If you want to look at your cervix, you will need to purchase a speculum. Metal or plastic speculums are available at many online retailers and are not very expensive. A note about speculums: Many people have negative associations with them, and for good reasons. So many people we know and have cared for have had traumatic experiences with speculums at the doctor's office where their provider didn't use appropriate informed consent during a speculum exam. If you have had a negative experience like this, it's not okay and we are sorry that this happened to you.

We also know it is possible to have positive, gentle, affirming experiences with speculums. This can happen with the right provider, at home with a friend or a partner, or by yourself. If you're interested in experimenting with and even redefining your relationship with speculums at home, we will walk you through the whole process, so it doesn't feel too scary or overwhelming.

Using a speculum is relatively simple, though it can take some practice. Be patient. Sometimes you need to try multiple times to be able to see the cervix, and you'll get more comfortable with practice. Below is a step-by-step guide for using a speculum to see your cervix. If you are not interested in using a speculum, skip to page 67.

HOW TO USE A SPECULUM

1. Choose the Right Space, and Gather Your Supplies

The best position for using a speculum is lying on your back on a comfortable, firm surface. If your bed is extra squishy, it will be challenging to get the speculum in the right position. If you have a firm mattress, that will be fine. Otherwise, you can use a yoga mat or lie on blankets on the floor.

Once you find the right spot in your home, gather your supplies: the speculum, lube, and a light. This can be the light on your phone or a headlamp (Ray and Marea use headlamps while they perform IUIs, which makes them look super cool). You may want to take a photo (with flash!) once you see your cervix, so have a phone ready. If you're doing this yourself, you'll need a mirror as well. Either a standing mirror or a hand mirror will work great.

2. Get into Position

You'll want a pillow for your head, as well as a firm pillow for underneath your lower back / sacrum. It works best if you feel like your butt is relaxed and hanging slightly off the pillow. We usually recommend putting a towel down under your butt in case some fertile cervical fluid or lube comes out while inserting the speculum or taking it out. Before lying down, take off your pants and underwear.

Once you get the pillow situated under your sacrum, put the soles of your feet together and relax your knees open in a butterfly position. We recommend putting a pillow under each of your knees for support. If butterfly position doesn't work for your body, bent knees with feet flat on the floor can work, too. If you're cold, or feel too exposed, you can cover yourself with a sheet or towel.

3. Slowly Insert the Speculum

Put a little bit of water-based lube or coconut oil on the outside of the bills of the speculum, and position the speculum sideways (so the handle is facing to one side of your body) and in line with your vagina / front hole. Some people spread open their labia before insertion to make sure it doesn't snag any pubic hair. If you're inserting it yourself, put it inside yourself slowly. If you're doing this with a partner, make sure you have clear, open communication and that you are talking about each movement before it happens.

With insertion, it's important to insert the speculum slightly downward, toward your sacrum, following the curve of the vagina / front hole. Many people don't realize that the vagina isn't straight—it actually curves downward, then upward, swooping toward the cervix, like a bowl. The speculum insertion will feel more comfortable if you follow this anatomical curve.

4. Rotate and Open the Speculum

Once inside, slowly rotate the speculum so the handle is facing either up or down (it doesn't matter), then open the speculum and lock it into place. Shine your light. If you can see your cervix, awesome! If you're doing this by yourself, it may take some time to get the hang of shining the light as well as holding the mirror at the right angle.

If you can't see your cervix, you can unlock the speculum and reposition it (try moving it even farther downward toward your sacrum—it's usually hiding there). If you still can't find it, try removing the speculum and then jumping up and down a few times before inserting the speculum again. Sometimes the gravity of jumping can help the cervix become more visible. If you *still* can't see your cervix, try making your hands into fists and placing them under your lower back, then tilting your pelvis upward slightly. This angle is a great trick for bringing the cervix into view.

This may sound complicated, but we promise that you'll get the hang of it quickly. Becoming familiar with your cervix is very helpful when trying to get pregnant, because your cervix will tell you exactly when you are ovulating. And again, if you just aren't into feeling or looking at your cervix, it's okay! Ray's favorite tracking tool, cervical fluid, is up next.

Cervical Fluid

Let's get intimate with our cervical fluid, aka cervical mucus! Checking your cervical fluid is easy to do, free, can be done internally or externally, and requires no additional tools. Tracking your cervical fluid offers additional information about your fertility and can pair nicely with feeling or looking at your cervix.

The cervix produces fluid, and the texture and quality of this fluid changes throughout the menstrual cycle. For most of the menstrual cycle, the fluid coming from the cervix is relatively dry, and sometimes sticky. As ovulation approaches, estrogen causes the cervical fluid to become more creamy in color and texture. Then, when ovulation is very close, it becomes watery and slick. Finally, during ovulation, cervical mucus is wet and stretchy, resembling an egg white. Cervical fluid dries up as soon as the ovulatory phase is over.

During the ovulatory phase, fertile mucus produced in the cervix acts as a highway for sperm, protecting it from the acidic environment of the vagina and helping it travel from outside the cervix to inside the uterus.

There are a few ways to check your cervical fluid. If you're feeling your cervical position with your fingers, you can check the mucus that remains on your fingers when you pull them out after you're done. You can also check your cervical mucus by dabbing your fingers or toilet paper at the opening of your vagina / front hole, then pinching the fluid between your fingers.

Some people notice very clear changes in their cervical fluid throughout their cycle, and others do not. If you don't notice significant changes throughout your cycle, you'll need to pay more attention to the other fertility signs. Sometimes changes in cervical fluid are hard to notice, and that is okay. Other times, if your other fertility signs don't line up, it could be an indication of ovulatory problems. It's helpful to know that taking allergy medication or decongestants can also negatively impact cervical mucus.

Basal Body Temperature (BBT)

Your basal body temperature, or BBT, is your body's temperature when you are fully at rest. And not just relaxed—*at rest* here means your body's temperature right upon waking up from a full night's sleep, before undertaking any physical activity or eating or drinking anything. Before ovulation, the human body averages between 97°F (36.1°C) and 97.5°F (36.4°C).[2] During ovulation, body temperature begins to rise, and forty-eight hours after ovulation, body temperature averages between 97.6°F (36.4°C) and 98.6°F (37°C)[3] and continues to stay elevated through the luteal phase due to the increase in the hormone progesterone, which is released by the ovaries at ovulation. That 0.5°F change in body temperature is the magic number and will tell you the exact day that you ovulated.

Tracking your BBT is a little more involved than some of the other fertility signs, but unlike tracking cervical mucus and cervical position and openness, which are used to *predict* ovulation, tracking your basal body temperature is a fascinating tool that allows you to *confirm* ovulation. In concert with other fertility signs, BBT can be a crucial piece in achieving a complete picture of ovulation timing.

When tracking your BBT, it's important to take your temperature with a digital basal body thermometer first thing in the morning, before getting up to pee or drinking water. Most people use a simple oral thermometer, but wearable temperature technology also exists. After taking your temperature, you can record your results each day on a BBT chart or app. You'll find a template in the appendix on page 276, or you can download one from www.babymakingforeverybody.com.

How to Figure Out Ovulation: The Cover Line

The key to noticing the temperature shift with ovulation is to create a cover line on a fertility chart. This is an imaginary line you draw on your BBT chart that denotes a separation between your pre-ovulatory and post-ovulatory temperatures and helps you visualize when ovulation has taken place. Ovulation occurs forty-eight hours before a 0.5°F temperature shift above the cover line.

Many apps will also calculate the cover line math so you don't have to (yay technology!), but if you choose to chart by hand, or want to know how the line is determined, here's what you do:

1. Identify a temperature that is at least 0.2°F higher than the previous six days.
2. Highlight those previous six days.
3. Find the highest of these six highlighted temperatures.
4. Draw a straight line across the entirety of your chart that is 0.1°F higher than the highest of the highlighted temperatures.

Let's look at a chart to see what this looks like:

ALEX'S BBT CHART

CYCLE DAY	1	2	3	4	5	6	7	8	9	10	11	12
	99	99	99	99	99	99	99	99	99	99	99	99
	9	9	9	9	9	9	9	9	9	9	9	9
	8	8	8	8	8	8	8	8	8	8	8	8
	7	7	7	7	7	7	7	7	7	7	7	7
	6	6	6	6	6	6	6	6	6	6	6	6
	5	5	5	5	5	5	5	5	5	5	5	5
	4	4	4	4	4	4	4	4	4	4	4	4
	3	3	3	3	3	3	3	3	3	3	3	3
	2	2	2	2	2	2	2	2	2	2	2	2
	1	1	1	1	1	1	1	1	1	1	1	1
BASAL BODY	98	98	98	98	98	98	98	98	98	98	98	98
TEMPERATURE (F)	9	9	9	9	9	9	9	9	9	9	9	9
	~~8~~	~~8~~	~~8~~	~~8~~	~~8~~	~~8~~	~~8~~	~~8~~	~~8~~	~~8~~	~~8~~	~~8~~
	7	7	7	7	7	7	7	(7)	7	7	7	7
	(6)	6	6	(6)	6	6	(6)	6	6	6	6	6
	5	(5)	(5)	5	5	(5)	5	5	5	(5)	(5)	5
	4	4	4	4	4	4	4	(4)	4	4	4	4
	3	3	3	3	(3)	3	3	3	3	3	3	(3)
	2	2	2	2	2	2	2	2	2	2	2	2
	1	1	1	1	1	1	1	1	1	1	1	1
	97	97	97	97	97	97	97	97	97	97	97	97
	9	9	9	9	9	9	9	9	9	9	9	9

So, on Alex's chart, we can see an obvious spike in BBT between days 15 and 16. That shift confirms that ovulation occurred forty-eight hours prior, on day 14. Knowing this information will support Alex to optimally time their inseminations when it's their time to conceive.

Does BBT Work for Everyone?

BBT tracking works well for people who have a regular sleep schedule (going to bed and waking up around the same time every day), aren't getting up regularly at night to care for a pet or a person, and like to pay attention to details. You need to have slept at least four

13	14	15	16	17	18	19	20	21	22	23	24	25	26	27	28	29	30
99	99	99	99	99	99	99	99	99	99	99	99	99	99	99	99	99	99
9	9	9	9	9	9	9	9	9	9	9	9	9	9	9	9	9	9
8	8	8	8	8	8	8	8	8	8	8	8	8	8	8	8	8	8
7	7	7	7	7	7	7	7	7	7	7	7	7	7	7	7	7	7
6	6	6	6	6	6	6	6	6	6	6	6	6	6	6	6	6	6
5	5	5	5	5	5	5	5	5	5	5	5	5	5	5	5	5	5
4	4	4	4	4	4	4	4	4	4	4	4	4	4	4	4	4	4
3	3	3	3	3	③	3	③	③	3	3	③	3	3	3	3	3	3
2	2	2	2	2	2	②	2	2	2	2	2	2	2	2	2	2	2
1	1	1	1	①	1	1	1	1	1	①	1	①	1	1	①	1	1
98	98	98	98	98	98	98	98	98	⑨⑧	98	98	98	⑨⑧	⑨⑧	98	98	98
9	9	9	9	9	9	9	9	9	9	9	9	9	9	9	9	9	9
8	8	8	8	8	8	8	8	8	8	8	8	8	8	8	8	8	8
7	7	7	⑦	7	7	7	7	7	7	7	7	7	7	7	7	⑦	7
6	⑥	6	6	6	6	6	6	6	6	6	6	6	6	6	6	6	6
5	5	⑤	5	5	5	5	5	5	5	5	5	5	5	5	5	5	5
④	4	4	4	4	4	4	4	4	4	4	4	4	4	4	4	4	4
3	3	3	3	3	3	3	3	3	3	3	3	3	3	3	3	3	3
2	2	2	2	2	2	2	2	2	2	2	2	2	2	2	2	2	2
1	1	1	1	1	1	1	1	1	1	1	1	1	1	1	1	1	1
97	97	97	97	97	97	97	97	97	97	97	97	97	97	97	97	97	97
9	9	9	9	9	9	9	9	9	9	9	9	9	9	9	9	9	9

consecutive hours for a BBT to be considered accurate, and it can also be thrown off if you're sick or travel on an airplane.

This method may not work as well for people who work night shifts, travel regularly, or who get up in the middle of the night to care for a pet or a child. Ray used this method while trying to conceive, but Marea, who had a two-year-old who didn't sleep through the night while she was trying to conceive (and is noticeably less detail-oriented than Ray), decided to rely on other signs to track her fertility.

If you get up at odd hours, don't adhere to a rigid schedule, or experience insomnia, you can either use wearable temperature technology or use other tracking methods that will give you more accurate information.

Luteinizing Hormone Levels and Ovulation Predictor Kits

You'll remember from our discussion of the menstrual cycle that luteinizing hormone is responsible for triggering the ovary to release an egg. Generally, the body starts producing this hormone one to three days prior to ovulation; production then surges when the egg is ready to be released. Once the surge occurs, LH stays elevated for about a day before dropping. People with PCOS may have LH in their body for longer, so this can be a less reliable tool (more about PCOS later in this chapter).

When LH surges in the body, an egg is typically released about twenty-four to thirty-six hours later. However, there is a large range when ovulation can occur, from six to fifty-six hours. Tracking LH levels is the final piece in tracking your fertility and figuring out optimal insemination timing, and we do this by using ovulation predictor kits. These simple, over-the-counter urine tests measure the amount of luteinizing hormone in your urine, and they're available online or at any drugstore.

Depending on the type of strips you use, your ovulation predictor kit will tell you with either a line or a symbol that you are in a pre-ovulatory phase. When the ovulation predictor strip shows a dark line or a "positive," it means that your LH is surging and that your body is preparing to release an egg.

We recommend starting to use ovulation predictor strips three to four days before your expected date of ovulation—which you should know thanks to your work tracking cervical position and mucus, and your BBT! It's helpful to test three times a day: once in the morning, once in the early afternoon, and once in the evening.

Why test so frequently? Because when determining ovulation, it is crucial to know when the beginning of the LH surge is occurring.

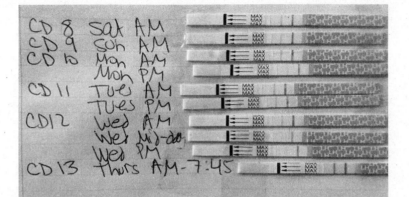

Once the surge happens, an OPK test will often remain positive for a day or two. If you test once a day in the evening and your LH surge happens in the morning, you will incorrectly identify when ovulation will occur and miss the optimal window for insemination.

It can be tempting to test more frequently than that, but we recommend limiting yourself to three times a day—your LH levels won't change much between those times, and we notice that some people can get a little obsessed peeing on the sticks. If testing in the middle of the day does not work with your schedule, test twice a day: first thing in the morning and in the evening.

In this photo, you can see the person's ovulation test strips evolve until they get a positive OPK on Thursday morning.

HELP! WHAT OPK TEST STRIPS SHOULD I BUY??

We get this question all the time, and the short answer is: Any OPK will do. The two most common options are the simple, cheaper version that show a purple line corresponding with LH levels, and the fancier, higher-tech Clearblue tests that feature a flashing smiley face while LH levels are rising and a solid smiley face when they reach the level high enough to induce ovulation. Many of our clients use the simpler (aka cheaper) OPKs as LH levels rise, and will time their insemination from the first positive reading. Others use the cheaper products when learning to track and then switch to Clearblue the months they are inseminating. If you're choosing this route, we recommend using your new product at least one month prior to your first insemination to alleviate any anxieties if the product works a little differently than what you're used to.

Okay, So How Do I Put All This Together?

Now you know how to feel or look at your cervix, check your cervical fluid, take your basal body temperature, and use ovulation predictor kits to track your LH levels. Tracking all four of these fertility signs helps you identify your ovulation, and in turn your optimal insemination timing.

So how do we put it all together? It may feel old school, but it's helpful to use a paper chart like the one below to track all your fertility signs. It not only helps you organize all your data, but also creates an easy visual of your fertile window. Below is an example of what this can look like, and you'll find a sample blank chart in the appendix on page 276, as well as on our website.

Your most fertile days are when your cervix is open, your cervical mucus is clear and stretchy, and right before your temperature rises. For example, in this chart, on days 15 and 16, we can see that the person's cervix is soft, their cervical mucus is egg-white / stretchy, and their temperature is low but about to rise. Plus, they got a positive OPK on the evening of day 14. From this information, we can assume that this person ovulates late on day 15 or early on day 16, so that's when they would plan their insemination.

TRACKING APPS

Okay, so even though we just recommended paper charts, we know most folks are going to use apps to track their cycle. That's okay! Just remember, use your app as a place to store data, not to time inseminations. Apps guess fertility windows and ovulation based on the previous month's data, *not* on your current cycle's data. As we've discussed there are a lot of factors that can affect ovulation timing month to month, so take your app's recommendation with a grain of salt and learn to track when you're ovulating instead.

This Is a Lot...Do I Have to Do It All the Time?

Once you have a clear sense of what day of your cycle you ovulate, you don't necessarily need to track all four signs. Some people like to keep track of each of their fertility signs, while others stick to their favorite two to give them all that information.

As we mentioned, it's helpful to spend at least two to three months putting all this information together before starting to inseminate, if possible, so that you can get used to tracking and interpreting it. If you're thinking that you may want to use your body to have a baby in the near future, start tracking now! Ideally, you'll get a sense of your fertile signs leading up to ovulation that will help you time your inseminations within about three months of tracking, but some people will require longer. After about seven months of tracking Ray was able to figure out that they ovulated eighteen hours after their LH surge, which allowed for more precise insemination timings. It's helpful to print out one chart per cycle and put them next to each other as a way to keep track of all the information.

Also, be gentle with yourself. Some people attempt to ace the fertility-tracking process by collecting all the data all the time, and

NAME: ALEX   **AGE:** 34   **MONTH:** March / April

CYCLE DAY	1	2	3	4	5	6	7	8	9	10	11	12	13	14	15	16	17
DATE	20	21	22	23	24	25	26	27	28	29	30	31	1	2	3	4	5

BASAL BODY TEMPERATURE (F) — recorded readings:

Cycle Day	1	2	3	4	5	6	7	8	9	10	11	12	13	14	15	16	17
Temp	97.6	97.5	97.6	97.6	97.3	97.5	97.6	97.4	97.7	97.5	97.6	97.3	97.4	97.6	97.5	97.7	98.1

	1	2	3	4	5	6	7	8	9	10	11	12	13	14	15	16	17
CERVICAL FLUID									S		S/C	C	CI	EW	EW	EW	S
CERVICAL POSITION				F	F	F		F			F				S	S	
CERVICAL OPENNESS				C	C	C		C			C				O	O	
OPK																	
INSEMINATION?																	

NOTES

- Day 1: Period, Day 1
- Day 2: Heavy flow
- Day 3: Heavy flow
- Day 8: slept in 30min
- Day 11: Little appetite in am
- Day 15: Feeling super tired
- Day 17: Little bit of sticky

2023	1	26	30	29
YEAR	CYCLE #	SHORTEST	LONGEST	CURRENT

18	19	20	21	22	23	24	25	26	27	28	29	30	31	32	33	34	35	36	37	38	39	40
6	7	8	9	10	11	12	13	14	15	16	17											
99	99	99	99	99	99	99	99	99	99	99	99	99	99	99	99	99	99	99	99	99	99	99
9	9	9	9	9	9	9	9	9	9	9	9	9	9	9	9	9	9	9	9	9	9	9
8	8	8	8	8	8	8	8	8	8	8	8	8	8	8	8	8	8	8	8	8	8	8
7	7	7	7	7	7	7	7	7	7	7	7	7	7	7	7	7	7	7	7	7	7	7
6	6	6	6	6	6	6	6	6	6	6	6	6	6	6	6	6	6	6	6	6	6	6
5	5	5	5	5	5	5	5	5	5	5	5	5	5	5	5	5	5	5	5	5	5	5
4	4	4	4	4	4	4	4	4	4	4	4	4	4	4	4	4	4	4	4	4	4	4
3	3	**3**	**3**	3	3	**3**	3	3	3	3	3	3	3	3	3	3	3	3	3	3	3	3
2	**2**	2	2	2	2	2	2	2	2	2	2	2	2	2	2	2	2	2	2	2	2	2
1	1	1	1	1	**1**	1	**1**	1	1	**1**	1	1	1	1	1	1	1	1	1	1	1	1
98	98	98	98	**98**	98	98	98	**98**	**98**	98	98	98	98	98	98	98	98	98	98	98	98	98
9	9	9	9	9	9	9	9	9	9	9	9	9	9	9	9	9	9	9	9	9	9	9
8	8	8	8	8	8	8	8	8	8	8	8	8	8	8	8	8	8	8	8	8	8	8
7	7	7	7	7	7	7	7	7	7	7	**7**	7	7	7	7	7	7	7	7	7	7	7
6	6	6	6	6	6	6	6	6	6	6	6	6	6	6	6	6	6	6	6	6	6	6
5	5	5	5	5	5	5	5	5	5	5	5	5	5	5	5	5	5	5	5	5	5	5
4	4	4	4	4	4	4	4	4	4	4	4	4	4	4	4	4	4	4	4	4	4	4
3	3	3	3	3	3	3	3	3	3	3	3	3	3	3	3	3	3	3	3	3	3	3
2	2	2	2	2	2	2	2	2	2	2	2	2	2	2	2	2	2	2	2	2	2	2
1	1	1	1	1	1	1	1	1	1	1	1	1	1	1	1	1	1	1	1	1	1	1
97	97	97	97	97	97	97	97	97	97	97	97	97	97	97	97	97	97	97	97	97	97	97
9	9	9	9	9	9	9	9	9	9	9	9	9	9	9	9	9	9	9	9	9	9	9
	S				S																	
	F	F		F	F	F	F			F												
	C	C		C	C	C	C			C												
										bad cramps and bloating	Period, Day 1											

it's easy to get overwhelmed and burned out by this approach. Try to integrate fertility tracking into your current lifestyle as much as possible, and give yourself permission to take breaks if needed. We are humans, after all, trying to make humans, and sometime human-ing is hard.

Words cannot explain how much I dislike cycle tracking. I began tracking my cycle in February 2020, thinking my partner and I would start inseminating that summer (ha!), and when the pandemic hit, I took a break and restarted tracking in July to start trying to conceive later that year.

My cycle is affected by stress and sleep loss, which makes sense and is an occupational hazard of midwifery. But when you're trying to figure out when you're ovulating, it is also maddening. I had months when just as I was about to ovulate, I'd go to a birth and lose sleep, so my ovulation would be delayed five to ten days. One month I peed on LH strips for twelve days before I got a positive surge.

My temperature data was inconsistent (mostly due to sleep loss). I decided to try a fancy thermometer that auto-synced with an app, and the weird gender stuff on the app made me feel like an alien. My unclear cover line made me feel like a failure. I loved interpreting temperature on other people's charts, but for my own chart it was wildly useless. I needed a friend to tell me to stop taking my temperature before I was willing to throw in the towel.

I was determined to do everything right. I took every supplement, started fertility acupuncture, did LH strips three times a day, and checked my cervix and cervical fluid two or three times a day. Unsurprisingly, I burned out quickly, stopped going to acupuncture, and when we had sperm bank delays (aka sperm jail) I tailspinned about having to be so attentive to my body and not drink eight cups of coffee a day forever. More than once I took a month off from trying just to smoke a cigarette and not feel like I was ruining everything.

Fertility can be a maddening process, and I became obsessed with the most exact timing. The truth is, tracking for longer periods of time does give you more data, and by seven months of good tracking I was able to determine that I ovulate closer to eighteen hours after my LH surge. The first time I timed my IUI with a shorter timing interval, I got pregnant.

That pregnancy didn't stick, but within two months of my miscarriage I felt like I understood my cycle again. I also deeply resented having to continue tracking. But when I considered the alternative—ultrasounds, blood work, medication (none of which I had insurance coverage for and also didn't guarantee any different outcomes)—tracking continued to make the most sense. —Ray

Troubleshooting Issues: What If My Fertile Signs Are All Over the Place?

Let's talk a little bit about people whose fertile signs are irregular or difficult to track. People who have irregular or no menstrual bleeding, experience very heavy or light periods, don't notice changes in their cervical mucus, don't get positive OPKs, or have irregular basal body temperatures may be experiencing anovulation (aka not ovulating).

Anovulatory cycles can happen for a variety of reasons, including PCOS and other high-androgen conditions, thyroid problems, high blood sugar, anemia, very low or high body weight, overexercise, eating disorders, extreme stress, certain cancers, medications, congenital anomalies, and lactation. If through tracking your fertile signs you notice that you may not be ovulating, we recommend you seek care with a provider who can offer lab tests and help you attain a clearer picture of what's happening in your body before beginning inseminations.

WHAT'S THE DEAL WITH PCOS?

Polycystic ovarian syndrome, or PCOS, is a condition in which the ovaries produce an abnormal amount of androgens, which are sex hormones typically found in bodies assigned male at birth. Some people notice symptoms of PCOS (facial hair, acne, abdominal weight distribution, elevated blood sugar, and irregular cycles, or ultrasound images of the ovaries with high follicle count), and some do not.

PCOS is *really* common, affecting 5 to 10 percent of people with uteruses.[4] PCOS is even more common in the LGBTQ+ community—with rates possibly as high as 38 percent.[5] The main issue with PCOS and fertility is that elevated levels of testosterone and metabolic stress from high blood sugar impede regular ovulation. If you have PCOS and have cycles lasting thirty-seven-plus days, you can learn more about regulating your cycle naturally on page 92, and can also use medications to stimulate ovulation and regulate blood sugar. If you aren't able to resume a cycle of twenty-one to thirty-six days within six months of using diet and lifestyle interventions—or you desire more guidance—we recommend seeing a fertility specialist.

Let's Talk About Sperm!

As we know, eggs are only half the equation for creating a pregnancy, and fertility is not the sole domain of people with uteruses. If your body makes sperm and you are trying to make a baby, we recommend testing your sperm for count and motility. You can get your sperm tested through your primary doctor, at your local sperm bank, or through a kit that you order online and then send to a lab for evaluation. It's a very simple process—you'll get all the information you need with one ejaculation.

If you (or your donor) have more than fifteen million motile sperm, you have the flexibility to choose whichever conception method is right for you. When the motile sperm count is under fifteen million but over ten million, utilizing some interventions like IUI is an effective method for conception. With a count of less than ten million, it's worth considering IVF. We'll go more in depth about these options in chapters 4 and 8.

How to Bank Your Sperm

People with sperm may want to bank their sperm for many reasons. We decided to include information on how to bank sperm in the fertility section of this book because depending on your unique fertility situation and baby-making plans, banking your sperm may be a great option for you. Some people are planning to initiate gender-affirming hormone therapy (GAHT) or gender-affirming surgery, and want to bank sperm prior to these procedures. Other hopeful parents may have found an egg donor they love, but don't yet have a surrogate to carry the pregnancy—in this case, they can donate sperm at a fertility clinic and then have the embryos stored until the right surrogate comes along. Or perhaps you are working with a sperm donor who lives on the other side of the country; in this case, you can bank their sperm and then have it shipped to another sperm bank closer to the person with a uterus who will be doing the inseminations.

Whatever the reason you choose to bank your (or your donor's) sperm, the first step is finding a facility close to your home. Sperm banking can happen at a fertility clinic or a sperm bank, and each option has different rates and storage fees. There is a newer option becoming available: banking your sperm from a home delivery kit. This can be a great alternative for people concerned about gender dysphoria when entering a clinic setting. We recommend calling a few clinics nearby to find the best rates in your area.

Banking sperm at a sperm bank starts off with an intake appointment, which typically includes a health history, a physical, and blood work. This checkup may be able to be waived depending on the clinic. After that comes the time to deposit a sperm sample. Typically, people are provided with a private room and a cup to leave the sample in. Bring items that will help you feel more comfortable providing sperm. Once the sample is provided, the sperm bank can freeze or wash it to be used for IUI or other fertility procedures (more details on this in the next chapter).

Supporting Your Fertility

Optimizing your fertility means optimizing your baby-creating chances, both for people planning to use their bodies to carry a pregnancy and for those planning to use their sperm or eggs in another person's body.

First, we want to say: You don't *have* to do anything to support your fertility. People create humans all the time without changing their diets or exercising for twenty minutes a day. For people with uteruses, if you are ovulating regularly and your body is offering the aforementioned signs of fertility, chances are high that you are indeed fertile and will get pregnant after some tries. If your body produces sperm and you have never taken GAHT, there is a 98 percent chance that your body produces sperm capable of creating a pregnancy.[6] If your body produces sperm and you are on GAHT, we recommend checking out chapter 5 for more information on fertility specifically for trans people.

If the following information feels stressful and overwhelming to you, please try not to take it all too seriously. We're including this section because many of our clients feel empowered when they take some agency over optimizing their fertility. While trying to conceive, it can feel like so much is out of our control—sometimes it feels good to take proactive steps, and they may actually help! Additionally, these fertility recommendations can also support having a healthy pregnancy and birth.

There is no magic, end-all-be-all for fertility support. Human bodies are complex organisms, and no recommendations will work equally well for everybody. When considering these ways to support your fertility, we encourage you to consider your whole-picture health—mental, physical, and spiritual—and to avoid any dietary or lifestyle changes that might do more harm than good. You know yourself, your body, your limits, and your needs best. As with everything: Take this information, filter it through the lens of your own experience and values, and trust yourself to make the best decision for you and your family.

Fertility Support for All Bodies

Food, Water, and Lifestyles That Support Fertility

Eat whole foods

When eating for fertility, we encourage our clients to focus on whole, unprocessed foods that are high in antioxidants, fiber, and healthy fats. Foods that are antioxidant-rich, such as vegetables, fruits, whole grains, and nuts, support your fertility by removing toxins from your body. Walnuts[7] and blueberries are especially high in antioxidants and—in our opinions—are super delicious.

It's also hugely supportive to eat healthy fats, which support a body's ability to ovulate as well as produce viable sperm.[8] Some of our favorite sources of healthy fats are avocados, nuts, and low-mercury fish like salmon and halibut.

Maintain your blood sugar

Studies have shown that eating regularly, particularly eating a big breakfast with protein, helps to regulate your hormone and blood sugar levels and therefore supports your fertility. This may be especially supportive for people with PCOS,[9] and has also been shown to support sperm health.[10] Blood sugar management supports all your body's systems and takes stress off your liver. In addition to a big breakfast, the easiest way to maintain your blood sugar is to eat protein with every meal and snack, and eat regularly so that your blood sugar levels don't get too high or too low.

Acupuncture for fertility

Acupuncture is a form of Chinese medicine that has amazing results for supporting fertility for people with all different types of bodies.[11] Getting regular acupuncture supports all your body's systems to function optimally, and acupuncturists are trained in methods of boosting fertility for people with testes and people with ovaries. Many cities around the US now have sliding-scale or low-fee community acupuncture clinics, and we highly recommend checking them out! Acupuncture is also a proven way to reduce stress, plus you can take a nap during your appointment.

WHAT'S THE DEAL WITH WEIGHT LOSS?

We live in an incredibly fatphobic society and a medical culture that equates weight with health and considers weight loss a cure for all medical issues, including PCOS (which is more common in the queer community—see page 80). This is BS. Focusing on weight loss instead of health practices is reductive and fatphobic. As queer midwives, we want to encourage folks to focus on getting protein with every meal, drinking lots of water, eating healthy fats and complex carbs throughout the day, finding movement that is enjoyable and *not* punishment, and connecting to community to find support and joy in your life instead of focusing on a number on a scale. Plus Size Birth (plussizebirth.com) is our go-to resource for all things fat-positive fertility, pregnancy, and birth.

Support your liver

Healthy liver filtration is a key to rockin' fertility. It's important, as much as possible, to reduce substances that make your liver work harder. Alcohol, cigarettes, energy drinks, very processed foods, and caffeine fall into this category. Of these, caffeine is often the one we get the most questions about. To clarify: No, you don't need to eliminate caffeine entirely, but try to reduce caffeine intake to one to two cups of coffee or other caffeinated beverages a day, and to stay hydrated. The same goes for alcohol: Minimize as much as possible, and stay hydrated while consuming alcohol. We know that all forms of smoking are pretty bad for fertility, so try to limit smoking or vaping whenever you can. When it comes to food, trans fats and processed foods are more work for your liver to process and can negatively impact the hormones that cause ovulation.

Stay hydrated

Being well hydrated supports fertility in so many ways. Drinking water facilitates the delivery of hormones throughout the body and lubricates your tissues and cells. For people with uteruses, staying hydrated increases production of cervical mucus. For those with sperm, it supports sperm quality and the quantity of semen produced per ejaculation.[12] Aim for half your body weight in ounces of water daily.

Exercise regularly, but not too intensely

Regular movement is so supportive to our bodies. It helps regulate our blood sugar levels, increase oxygenation, improve our moods, and regulate hormones—all things that support our fertility. We recommend some kind of regular physical activity while trying to conceive, such as walking, cycling, lifting, yoga, or dancing three to five times a week. Just be aware that intense exercise can be associated with lowering fertility levels in some people.

Navigating Stress When Trying to Conceive

Let's face it: Trying to conceive can be stressful and anxiety provoking. And unfortunately, there is some evidence that high stress may negatively affect fertility[13] for people with all reproductive organs.[14] If you struggle with stress and anxiety while trying to conceive, you are not alone. Luckily there are some helpful techniques for reducing stress and anxiety that can be very supportive to your trying-to-conceive (TTC) process and overall well-being. These are some of our favorites to recommend to clients—feel free to pick and choose the options that resonate the best with you.

Find a support group or a friend you can talk to about your experiences

It's challenging to navigate trying to conceive alone, especially as an LGBTQ+ person and/or prospective solo parent. If possible, find a support group in your area or online for people you relate to who are TTC and lack all the components to create a pregnancy. We offer ideas of where to find online support groups on page 297. And if you're in the Philly area, you're always welcome at Ray's picnics! You can find details for Philly gatherings on Ray's practice Instagram: @refugemidwifery. If groups aren't your thing, try to find at least one friend who can be your buddy during this process.

Meditation and mantras

In times of stress, Marea has found it helpful to choose a phrase or two that combats whatever anxiety or hardship she is experiencing and say it over and over. Something like, "This is going to pass." Or "I am safe and healthy, and my baby will come when the time is right." The words are less important than the feeling they impart. When the anxiety or emotional pain surfaces, her mantras help diffuse the stressful energy and turn it into something less destabilizing (most of the time).

This works with meditation as well. Practicing meditation, even just for five minutes, can do wonders for calming your mind and your nervous system. Sit down in a comfortable seated position, set a timer on your phone, and practice putting your attention on your in-and-out breath. There are also many wonderful guided meditations on YouTube, Spotify, and Insight Timer, and nonprofit organizations like Insight LA that offer free meditation classes online or in person.

Talk to a therapist

Having a skilled mental health professional to support you while trying to conceive is essential for many of our clients and can vastly improve your emotional and mental experience. We recommend trying to find a therapist who has experience supporting people through their TTC process, and who is 100 percent supportive of your identity and family formation choices. Some fertility clinics have reproductive psychologists who are skilled at counseling people during this time in their lives, and some are covered under certain insurance plans. There are also therapists who focus on supporting people in their family-building process, and may specialize in working with LGBTQ+ people and solo parents. We offer suggestions for finding the right healthcare professional for you on page 127.

Connect with nature and move your body

Scientists have learned that being in nature reduces stress and induces feelings of happiness (shocking!).[15] Even for city people like Ray who hate hiking, a walk around the neighborhood or sitting by the river can be a simple reset. So here is a reminder to go hug a tree (or not), get into or near a body of water, or look up at the moon. In moments of stress, even just a ten-minute walk in fresh air can make a huge difference to mental health.

Create ritual

> In the beginning, my wife and I did as many things as we could think of to prepare to welcome a child into our family. Our approach will probably resonate with many people who need assistance conceiving and/or have a tendency toward detailed family planning. We saved money for years and made a budget; we received generous sharing from queer friends and kids of queer parents about their journeys in family making; we talked with straight friends who went through fertility treatments; we read books; we consulted with queer midwives and lesbian doctors; we talked through many different scenarios; we watched documentaries; we made a conception game plan. We felt as ready as we could be. But looking back, if I could redo the beginning of our conception journey, I would have started with a ritual. —Nikiko Masumoto

Ritual has a powerful way of creating containers around our experiences and supporting us spiritually to keep our intentions and energy aligned. If you're not sure where to start with ritual, keep it simple. You can write your intentions down and put them near or in a bowl of clean water. You can write your fears down and then (safely) burn them to let them go. If your culture has rituals marking life change, try them. Whatever type of ritual helps you connect with yourself and your intentions will be supportive on your journey.

We did a really sweet conception ritual before the embryo transfer, conceptualized by my friend Aquia. Part of being queer is making what we need. We need more conception rituals—it feels like our birthright and even obligation as queers to smash heteropatriarchy and privatization / nuclear-family-ness whether we are partnered or not. This is a huge threshold for us that is important to mark.

The night before the transfer we did a visualization of my womb and uterus together that was beautiful and hilarious. Then we shared blessings, and everyone was asked to put their love and intentions into a bowl of water by or under their bed the night before and to dream all things queer and sticky and fertile. In the morning, everyone took that water and used it to water a seed they planted. —Kate Shapiro

Minimize screen time

Many studies are showing that the more time we spend in front of screens, the higher our stress levels become.[16] When trying to conceive, it can be tempting to follow all the TTC pages, watch all the YouTubes the internet has to offer, read all the articles, and so on. If this helps you feel less alone in the process, we support you—to an extent. Make sure to also take time away from your screen to connect with yourself without technology getting in the way.

> At some point in our conception process, I asked my partner to join all the LGBTQ TTC Facebook groups I was in so they could be stressed out with me about all the information. They suggested instead that I unfollow the groups that were giving me anxiety, which turned out to be a better plan. —Til

---

Now let's focus on things that folks can do to support their fertility. We'll start with recommendations specific to AMAB (assigned male at birth) people, and then talk about AFAB (assigned female at birth) people beginning on page 92.

Fertility Support for People with Testes

Nutrition and Supplements

The antioxidants found in fruits and vegetables have a very positive effect on fertility. Specifically, eating cruciferous vegetables (broccoli, kale, cabbage) and vegetables with beta-carotene (carrots) and tomatoes for their lycopene will help cleanse your body of toxins and support it to better utilize nutrients to produce healthy sperm. Some vitamins, herbs, and antioxidant supplements have also been shown to have positive effects on sperm counts. A study from the Department of Medical Pathophysiology of the University of Rome revealed some supplements that improve sperm counts.[17] We know we've provided an overwhelming number of options on this list, so we put a * next to our favorites.

Antioxidants

- N-acetyl-cysteine: 600 mg/day*
- CoQ10: 400mg/day*
- L-carnitine: 2–3g/day
- Acetyl-L-carnitine: 3g/day

- Glutathione: 600mg/day
- Astaxanthin: 16mg/day
- Lycopene: 4–8mg/day*

Herbs

- Ashwagandha: 675mg/day*
- Tribulus: 250mg/day
- Maca: 1500–3000mg/day

Vitamins

- Vitamin C + vitamin E: 1g/day
- Folic acid: 5mg/day*
- Zinc: 66mg/day*
- Selenium: 100mg/day

There are no standardized protocols of exactly what to take in what combination for improving sperm quality, nor do we think you should take twenty vitamins a day—it's unsustainable financially and emotionally. Instead, focus on getting one to three nutrients from each category, ideally in a combined supplement so you're taking fewer pills. That can be a multivitamin with zinc, folate, and vitamins C+E; an herbal supplement with Tribulus and maca; and a CoQ10 or lycopene combo or another mixed antioxidant.

When looking into which antioxidants might be right for you, check out the other conditions they address and pick the one that best fits your specific health needs. For instance, N-acetyl-cysteine helps regulate blood sugar, so if you have diabetes or struggle with blood sugar highs and lows, that would be a good fit.

Avoid Human-Made Estrogens

There are tons of sources of synthetic estrogens in our environment that are important to avoid if you are trying to increase your sperm health. Minimize exposure to hot plastics that come with food, bath or face products that contain parabens, and certain foods that have parabens added as a preservative.

Avoid Hot Tubs

Submerging the testicles in hot water negatively affects sperm health, so make sure to avoid hot baths and hot tubs while you're trying to boost sperm health. Hot showers do not have the same effect on sperm count because the core temperature of the testicles is not increasing.

Promote Blood Flow to Testicles

Wear loose underwear and avoid tucking if possible. Allowing oxygen-rich blood to flow through your testicles supports sperm cell maturation.

Fertility Support for People with Uteruses

Prenatal or Multivitamin with Folate, Not Folic Acid

Multivitamins provide our bodies with micronutrients that support our fertility. It's especially important to find a multivitamin with folate, not folic acid (the synthetic form of folate), since many people can't absorb folic acid, and if this is the case, it can actually negatively impact your fertility. The recommendation is 400mcg/day when trying to conceive.

Maca

Maca is a root native to South America that is rich in vitamins and minerals, supports your hormones, reduces stress within the body, helps to regulate your blood sugar, and has been shown to support fertility for AFAB folks.[18]

Vitex

Vitex, or chasteberry, is an herb native to Asia and the Mediterranean area that is well known for supporting the hormones involved in regulating the menstrual cycle.[19] It is a low-risk herbal intervention for regulating your menstrual cycle, and its uses for fertility have been well documented for centuries. We know many people with irregular cycles who, after taking vitex in capsule or tincture form for three months, develop a more regular cycle of menstruation and ovulation.

CoQ10

CoQ10 is an antioxidant that naturally occurs within our bodies. There is evidence[20] suggesting that taking a CoQ10 supplement supports egg production and improves fertility outcomes. We recommend 200mg a day.

Vitamin D

Some studies have shown that people with normal vitamin D levels have higher[21] rates of conception and live births, and since many of us are inside for larger portions of the day than our ancestors were, it's common to have low vitamin D levels in our society. It can be helpful to test your vitamin D levels to determine whether or not to start taking a supplement. Generally, we recommend 2000 IU a day. Since vitamin D is a fat-soluble vitamin and people can take too much, we recommend determining the ideal supplementation levels with your healthcare provider through a simple blood test.

Omega-3s

Omega-3s are fatty acids (aka healthy fats) that can improve[22] the quality of follicles and increase chances of embryo formation and implantation. Omega-3s can be found in fish, shellfish, nuts, seeds, and vegetables, but you can also consume them in supplement form. A dose of 1500 IU/day has been shown to support fertility.

———————

You can find some of our favorite vitamins at www.babymaking foreverybody.com. When selecting vitamins, we're big fans of food-based supplements—meaning that the vitamin is extracted from plants instead of made in a lab.

———————

Phew, that's a lot about fertility and how to support it! We hope that we were able to deliver this information in ways that help you feel empowered and not like you need to throw this book out the window. It's also okay if you're a little overwhelmed: This is a lot of information about very loaded parts of the body. Some people need to take a break at this point and think about something other than fertility for a hot minute. If this is you, take all the time you need.

In our next chapter, we'll talk about how to apply this information to create a pregnancy.

CHAPTER 4

Getting Pregnant: From Turkey Baster to Test Tube and Everything in Between

Hopeful solo parents and LGBTQ+ people are often "trying" to get pregnant long before their first insemination. Doing research, making decisions around where to get the genetic material you need, saving money, finding providers to help make a baby—it's a lot! Whether you've already chosen your sperm or egg source or are still gathering information, you're probably wondering about how to put everything together to conceive a baby, and that's where this chapter takes us next: We've got our why, and our what—it's time to talk about *how*.

We'll start with the most DIY conception options and move step by step from the least to most medicalized processes, reviewing the insemination logistics for ICI, IUI, and IVF (including co-IVF), the success rates of each method, as well as what to consider when choosing a conception method.

Our goal in this chapter is twofold: First, to empower you with the information you need to decide which insemination method makes the most sense for you, and second, to support you in maximizing the efficiency of your chosen conception method.

The first two sections of this chapter are addressed to folks with available eggs and uteruses in their relationship, but are also applicable to people with sperm using traditional surrogacy. The last section on IVF includes information for people with or without a uterus in their relationship.

One last word to the wise before we dive in: At this point in your process, you are *so close* to making a baby, and you may be feeling nervous and excited (or myriad other emotions). The cost and planning that go into LGBTQ+ and solo parent conception can make people feel a lot of pressure to get everything perfect, and we want to remind you that there's no "perfect" when it comes to making a baby. There are, however, ways to bring your full selves, your priorities, and your community into the process, and we hope this chapter can equip you with all the information you need to decide how you would like to grow your family with confidence and ease.

Before You Start: Know Your Fertility Window

Conception, the moment when a sperm cell fertilizes an egg cell (that later implants in the uterus), can happen in a body in the fallopian tube in the twelve to twenty-four hours after ovulation or, in the case of IVF, in a fertility clinic lab. Before you start trying to get pregnant, if you're using ICI or IUI, you'll need a good sense of the fertile window of the person who is planning to carry the pregnancy—aka when the egg is about to be released—to know when to time inseminations.

From your work in chapter 3, hopefully you have a good sense of when in your cycle you ovulate. (If you need a refresher on how to calculate this, head back to "Okay, So How Do I Put All This Together" on page 74). While there isn't a way to know the exact moment of ovulation with 100 percent certainty, the good news is that we don't need to: When it comes to timing inseminations, you'll be targeting something called the fertile window.

In the days prior to ovulation, estrogen levels rise and cervical mucus changes to assist with conception. The egg-white fluid acts as a superhighway for sperm to enter the uterus. Fresh sperm can live in egg-white cervical fluid for up to three to five days. Frozen sperm generally live up to twelve hours, possibly up to twenty-four.

By charting the time when the cervix is the highest and most open, when there is the most cervical fluid, and when it stops, then putting that information together with LH strips and temperature spikes (again, for a refresher, head back to chapter 3), you can identify the ideal window of time to inseminate.

For example: If we have a client who, eight hours after getting a positive OPK, experiences mittelschmerz (pain/cramping in the ovaries during ovulation), and their temperature increases above the cover line the next day, we will recommend inseminating about eight hours after positive OPK. If somebody has a positive OPK, but then thirty-six hours later has tons of ovulatory cervical mucus and a very open cervix, we will recommend waiting until then to inseminate. Again: Humans are not robots! And this is why it's helpful to use all available data to inform our insemination timing.

As we age, the window between peak luteinizing hormone and the moment our bodies release the egg tends to get shorter. So, while we generally recommend IUI twenty-four hours after the positive OPK for our clients under age thirty-five, for clients closer to forty we have noticed that IUI closer to twelve to eighteen hours after the positive OPK is often more ideal.

OUR GENERAL INSEMINATION TIMING RECOMMENDATIONS

Under 35 with regular fertile signs: Inseminate 24 hours after the positive OPK.

Over 35 with regular fertile signs: Inseminate 12 to 24 hours after the positive OPK.

Still not able to reliably identify your ovulation after tracking your fertile signs for at least three months? Consider a consultation with midwives or a fertility clinic.

Once you and your partner(s) or surrogate have a clear idea of the fertile window you'll be working with, you're ready to acquire sperm and start inseminations!

Not a Turkey Baster: ICI

The simplest, cheapest, and most accessible form of insemination is intracervical insemination, also known as ICI. ICI is the process of inserting an unwashed semen sample as close to the cervix as possible at or right before ovulation so that the sperm can swim up through the cervix and fertilize an egg inside the fallopian tubes. You can use either fresh or frozen semen for ICI, though there are notable differences in timing and rates of conception for the two. The benefits of ICI include that it is initially affordable and accessible, you have more control over the process, and it doesn't require a speculum or a provider so individuals can get pregnant in their own bed, and can, if applicable, have a more intimate experience with their partner.

Most individuals who pursue ICI at home do so without a healthcare provider. This method is commonly joked about as the "turkey baster" method, but anyone who's actually seen a semen sample knows that a turkey baster is *way* too big a tool for this job. In reality, ICI uses a needle-less one- or three-milliliter syringe that you can buy at any drugstore for less than a dollar. Some people also forgo the syringe altogether and use a menstrual cup or a cervical cap to put the semen near the cervix. We will describe both methods in the following section.

WHAT HAPPENS DURING CONCEPTION ANYHOW?

When a sperm cell fertilizes an egg cell, the fertilized egg starts multiplying its cells, and then is called blastocyst. About six days after the blastocyst forms, it reaches the uterus and begins to implant inside the uterine walls.[1] It takes three to four days for the clump of cells to fully attach to the oxygen-rich uterine lining, and as the blastocyst creates an outer layer of cells that will become the placenta, it becomes an embryo. The fertilized egg releases hormones to prevent the period from occurring. If the blastocyst is formed in a lab during IVF, it is placed in the uterus after growing for five days.

How to Inseminate at Home

First, pull back the plunger on the syringe to add a little air, and then draw up the semen sample into a syringe. The person who's trying to get pregnant should empty their bladder, then lie down wherever they would like to do the insemination with a towel under their bottom. The person doing the inseminating—could be yourself, a partner, or a friend—gently inserts the syringe inside the vagina / front hole as deep as possible, then plunges the contents of the syringe inside the body and removes the syringe. Some sperm will spill out—this is okay. Only 1 percent of sperm that goes in a body makes it through the cervix into the uterus, and people still get pregnant.

Some folks also utilize a cervical cap as part of their insemination. A cervical cap is a soft, disposable menstrual cup, and its purpose is to hold the semen at the cervix during the day of insemination so that more sperm have an opportunity to swim up into the uterus. One study from 1986 found that heterosexual couples who were trying to conceive who used a cervical cap after intercourse got pregnant faster than couples who didn't.[2] It hasn't been studied since; however, it's a low-cost, simple intervention that may increase the chance of conception slightly by allowing the sperm to sit directly at the cervix

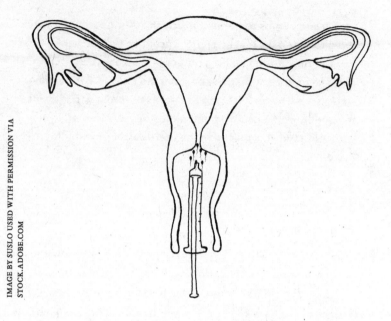

IMAGE BY SUSLO USED WITH PERMISSION VIA STOCK.ADOBE.COM

for as long as you leave it inside. If you choose to use a cervical cap, we suggest removing it after about twelve hours.

Insemination with a cervical cap can be done two ways. In the first, you use the syringe method described above and then fold the cap in half and insert it all the way in until you can feel the edge of the cervix around it. The second option is to pour the semen directly into the cap before inserting it into the body around the cervix. You can also use a menstrual cup. If this is your first time inserting a cervical cap or a menstrual cup, we recommend practicing before your first insemination, since it can be a bit tricky until you get the hang of it.

After the sperm is inside the body, many people opt to lie down for fifteen to twenty minutes to help bathe the cervix in sperm. Many midwives (like us) also suggest that folks try to have an orgasm, if this is an option for you. Orgasms contract the uterus and cause the cervix and uterus to pull upward, and these movements help suck sperm up into the uterus.

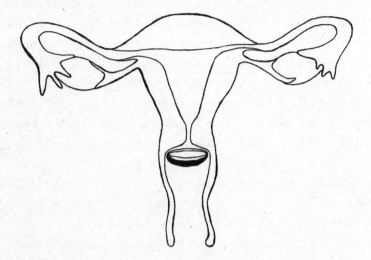

Each time we tried to conceive at home, things got easier and easier. However, the roller coaster of emotions waiting two weeks to test, being hopeful, then getting let down was not easy at all. Luckily, the third time was a charm. I had gotten the pregnancy tests that said the words PREGNANT or NOT PREGNANT, so there would be no mistake. When the word PREGNANT came on the screen that morning before work, I couldn't believe it. I didn't feel ready and I was nervous to get too excited too quickly. —Sauce Leon

As with all methods of conception, though, timing is essential. The ideal time to perform ICI differs whether you're using fresh or frozen sperm. Let's take a closer look at both options.

ICI with Fresh Sperm

If you have a known donor providing fresh sperm samples, or you are providing sperm for your traditional surrogate, fresh inseminations can be performed throughout the fertile window, starting when you or your surrogate has fertile cervical mucus and up until about twenty-four hours after the LH surge. When doing one insemination per cycle, the best timing for most people is the day of the LH surge to about twelve to twenty-four hours after the surge. With multiple inseminations, it's important to space out each ejaculation to allow time to rebuild an optimal sperm count. If people ejaculate multiple times during the course of a day, their sperm count will be low in each sample, meaning each insemination will be less effective. Higher sperm count yields the best chance of conception, therefore, having a longer gap between each ejaculation (at least twenty-four but ideally forty-eight hours) or just one, well-timed insemination is better than doing a ton of inseminations too close together.

The chance of conception with ICI with fresh sperm is the same as a heterosexual couple having intercourse during ovulation, which generally ranges from 15 to 20 percent per cycle. This number, for most people, decreases with age. We find this chart helpful for visualizing ideal timing for ICI. These are the conception rates for heterosexual couples based on the day they had intercourse near ovulation:[3]

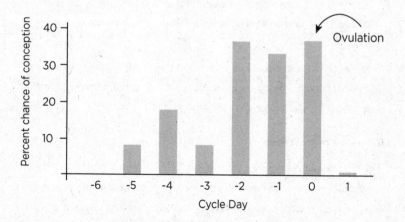

HOW TO COLLECT A FRESH SPERM SAMPLE

The person contributing sperm ejaculates into a clean, dry container with an airtight lid. Once the sperm sample is outside the body, it needs to stay at or near body temperature until it is put inside the body of the person trying to get pregnant. This can be done by holding the container in your underarm or between your legs. The sooner you can get to a location to inseminate, the better. We recommend not letting the sperm be outside the body for more than one hour.

We were nervous about trying to inseminate at home on our own for so many reasons—it was a pre-vaccine COVID world, we didn't know anyone else who had done an insemination at home, and we weren't sure how to logistically handle our donor's and our privacy. My partner took on the role of researching how to inseminate most effectively and learned a lot more about semen than she ever thought possible along the way! Before I ovulated, she ordered the suggested needle-less syringes and practiced sucking liquids into the syringe. —Abbey Nova

ICI with Frozen Sperm

The difference when using frozen sperm for ICI is that the timing window of insemination is much narrower. While fresh sperm can live for three to five days in the fallopian tubes, frozen sperm lives for about twelve hours, possibly up to twenty-four hours. Because previously frozen sperm doesn't live as long as fresh, the chance of conception with frozen sperm ICI is 5 to 10 percent per cycle.

If you do choose to perform ICI with frozen sperm, precise timing is essential. The ideal insemination timing is the beginning of the window when your egg is released. As providers, we generally recommend doing intrauterine inseminations (IUI) when using frozen sperm because it has double the success rate of ICI with frozen sperm.[4]

THAWING A FROZEN SPERM SAMPLE

Frozen sperm comes in an obscenely large tank that looks like a rocket ship. Leave it inside its rocket ship in your house until it is time for your insemination. When it's time, cut the plastic zip tie securing the lid, and then carefully pull the lid off. Using a towel or a potholder, pull the metal hook that's hanging on the edge of the lid up and out; that will be attached to the tube holding your sperm. It will be very cold! And very tiny! You will have a moment of *How the %$#)! is this tiny thing so much $$$$?!?!*

Very carefully remove the sperm from the holder with a towel or potholder. If you touch the liquid nitrogen with your bare skin, it will burn you. You can then defrost the sample one of two ways:

- Swirl the tube in a cup of room-temperature water. (*Not hot!* The water should feel about body temperature—test it on your wrist to be sure.) Keep the vial submerged until it's liquid.
- Put the sperm vial on the counter for ten to fifteen minutes.[5]

Once the sperm is defrosted, some people will put the container in an armpit for three to five minutes to warm the sperm up to body temperature, and some people won't. Both techniques have been studied and are okay!

As we mentioned earlier, the benefits of ICI include that it is affordable, simple, and potentially a very mellow and intimate experience. ICI with fresh sperm has high conception rates averaging 15 to 20 percent per cycle, possibly a little higher when inseminations are very well timed. The cons of ICI primarily have to do with frozen sperm. While it is cheaper to order frozen sperm to your home and inseminate yourself, the conception rates are low, ranging from 5 to 10 percent per cycle. With ICI with fresh sperm, the cons include considerations around logistics, donor contracts, legal navigation of stopping a donor's parental rights after birth, awkwardness surrounding the sperm donation, and protection from STIs, which requires trust and a relationship with your donor. If ICI doesn't seem quite right, or if you've already tried a few ICIs and want to up your chances of conception, you can consider doing an intrauterine insemination (IUI) with the help of a provider.

Start using terms and direct language like *pregnancy journey*, *fertility process*, *cycle where I didn't get pregnant*, and *insemination*. Don't use terms/euphemisms like *infertility*, *failed IUI*, *unsuccessful*, and *trying*. They are total downers.

Months ago, a close friend of mine, checking in on my process, sent me a text: "When's your next insem?" I loved the term *insem* so much that now I use it whenever I can. Even though this process can be extremely emotionally taxing, and words are practically meaningless when you find out you're not pregnant for the fifth time(!!), they actually do influence and shape the emotional tenor of your experience, especially when describing it to others (family, friends, et cetera), so find language that makes you laugh or feel radical or brings you joy. —Ellie Lobovits

IUI—When Sperm Hitch a Ride to the Fallopian Tubes

Ray and Marea both used IUI in their conception journeys, and it's another common and effective go-to insemination method for our communities in creating pregnancies. IUI was originally developed in fertility clinics as a treatment for heterosexual couples where there was an infertility issue in the sperm, a cervical issue blocking conception, or an unknown cause of infertility, but it's now commonly used with LGBTQ+ and solo parents by choice because the conception rates are much higher than ICI when using frozen sperm.[6]

In broad strokes, IUI is the process of inserting a washed sperm sample directly into the uterus for the purposes of conception. The way it works is that your provider thaws a washed sperm sample, then draws it into a sterile IUI catheter. Once the sperm is ready, the person receiving the IUI lies down and a speculum is inserted into the vagina / front hole to visualize the cervix. The catheter is then inserted through the cervix into the uterus, where the sperm is deposited at the top or fundus of the uterus, near the fallopian tubes. After the sperm is inside the uterus, the catheter comes out, and then the speculum comes out. It's typical to stay lying down for fifteen to twenty minutes afterward, because studies have found that this period of rest slightly increases the chance of conception.[7]

WHAT DOES IUI FEEL LIKE?

The most uncomfortable part of the IUI procedure, for most people, is the insertion of the speculum. Once the speculum is placed and the provider can see the cervix, the insertion of the sterile catheter, for most folks, doesn't cause pain or discomfort. Since the catheter is so thin and the cervix is open during ovulation, it usually goes inside very easily.

Some people do feel some mild cramping while the sperm sample is inserted into the uterus, but the experience is generally pretty smooth and comfortable.

Most IUIs occur in fertility clinics, but if there is a midwife who offers home or office IUI in your area, that can be a great option (and much cheaper depending on your insurance coverage or lack thereof). The timing for IUI is guided by cycle tracking and LH strips or blood work and ultrasounds. There are some costs to IUI in addition to frozen sperm. IUI with a midwife, at the time of this writing, ranges from $250 to $450 per try. At a fertility clinic, IUI can range from $500 to $3,000, depending on monitoring and medications used. Even though it can be expensive, it is essential to have a trained provider do the IUI for you, because without the use of sterile technique there is a risk of developing a uterine infection.

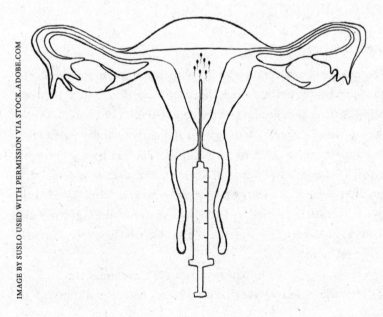

WHAT IS SPERM WASHING?

A fresh semen sample contains seminal fluid and sperm cells. Seminal fluid's job is to protect sperm cells from the acidic environment of the vagina, and once deposited in a body, sperm cells swim up the cervix into the uterus, leaving the seminal fluid behind. Sperm washing is the process of separating seminal fluid from sperm so that just the sperm cells can be placed inside the uterus. Seminal fluid contains bacteria and other materials that are dangerous to place directly into the uterus. During ICI, the cervix does that job of filtering out the non-sperm matter from the seminal fluid, but in IUI we bypass the cervix entirely.

ICI can be done with both ICI- and IUI-ready vials of frozen sperm. However, if you are planning to do IUI, you can only use sperm that is washed and IUI-ready, unless your clinic or midwife washes the ICI vial for you.

Success Rates

The chance of conception with IUI with frozen sperm is generally 12 to 16 percent per cycle, though the range can be found to be between 9 and 20 percent depending on the data source.[8] The conception rate does generally decline with age, so IUI success under twenty-five years old is about 19 percent per cycle, whereas by age forty it's typically closer to 9 percent.[9] In Ray's practice, they have found that about 15 percent of clients get pregnant per cycle. This makes sense to us, because in midwifery-led IUI we are not working with folks who have a known fertility issue—just those who lack sperm in their life or relationship.

The average number IUIs it takes to achieve pregnancy is four. It's typically been thought that if you don't conceive within four to six IUIs, it's less likely to work and it's time to move on to different fertility interventions. However, most of the data about IUI incorporates only heterosexual couples with infertility seeking treatment. More recent studies suggest that conception rates with IUI continue to increase for queer couples until ten IUIs.[10] Since IUI is one-fortieth of the cost of IVF, this newer data suggests it could be worthwhile to try more than four IUIs. As always, this is a personal choice that depends on many factors, including your timeline for getting pregnant, financial means, and emotional experience.[11]

Timing IUI

The most ideal timing for IUI is to insert the sperm right when the egg is beginning to be released from the ovary at ovulation, so the egg has a maximum amount of time to meet the sperm (reminder: Eggs are viable for twelve to twenty-four hours).[12] As we already mentioned, IUI can be timed by tracking your fertility signs and using knowledge about your body plus OPK test strips. In a fertility clinic setting, IUI can also be timed by blood tests, ultrasounds, and medication. Medication called a trigger shot can also be used to time IUI (don't worry, we will talk more about medicated cycles on page 112).

Most typically, the egg is released from the ovary twenty-four to thirty-six hours after the LH surge (although again, the wide range of normal is six to fifty-two hours). The most common timing for IUI based on ovulation predictor kits is to do the insemination twenty-four hours after the first positive reading.[13] Remember, by the time you see that the LH surge is happening on an OPK, it has already started. When tracking for home IUI, we recommend testing with OPKs three times a day.

There can be a bigger range of ovulation timing from the LH surge, and the only way to know that with your own tracking is to use all the fertility-tracking signs to determine when you ovulate in relation to the LH surge. Some people ovulate a little bit later, so timing the insemination at thirty-six or forty-eight hours might make sense. We have both found in practice (and research also suggests) that folks closer to age forty tend to ovulate in a slightly shorter window, so performing an IUI twelve to eighteen hours after the LH surge might give you a greater chance at success. To learn what your body's normal is so that you can best time insemination, use as many of the tracking methods that we outline in chapter 3 as possible, and track for at least three months.

Not all cycles give really clear data. If you are a person whose cycles do not give clear information about ovulation, you feel the pressure of age, you do not want to track for months at home, or you would feel more comfortable using external medical tools like ultrasounds, blood work, and trigger shots to time insemination, you may be best be served by working with a fertility clinic.

Some fertility clinics have clients track their cycles with LH strips to time insemination, but many monitor ovarian follicle size and hormone levels with vaginal ultrasounds and blood tests for the days leading up to ovulation. External monitoring tools aren't fail-proof; it is possible to miss ovulation when utilizing fertility clinic tools. And even if you're using a fertility clinic, having a sense of when you ovulate is helpful to guide when to start monitoring in the clinic.

IUI and Fresh Sperm

By and large, for solo parents and LGBTQ+ people, IUI is performed with frozen sperm that was washed for insemination. Some people want to use fresh sperm for IUI, which can happen if the semen is washed right before the procedure. We don't have clear data on comparative success rates between frozen and fresh sperm samples with IUI, but it makes sense to assume that since fresh sperm generally has higher sperm counts and more motility, IUI may work slightly better with it.

IUI with fresh sperm is almost exclusively used as a treatment for heterosexual couples with infertility, so we don't know exactly how their data translates to queer and single bodies. Ray tells their clients that for people without infertility, conception rates for IUI with fresh sperm are possibly a bit higher than fresh sperm ICI conception rates, but it also adds cost and logistical challenges to what could otherwise be a free, DIY insemination procedure. Due to clinic rules and FDA regulations around infectious disease testing for people not partnered with their sperm donor, this option may not be available in your area.

> We started trying with home IUI with a midwife, and after six tries, one pregnancy, and one miscarriage switched to ICI with a local donor. I really preferred ICI; it was a lot more comfortable for my partner, we didn't need anyone's help to do it so the experience was more intimate, and I was able to be more involved in getting her pregnant.
> —Asher

How Many Inseminations Should I Do per Cycle?[14]

Many of our clients wonder if doing more than one insemination per cycle will increase their chance of conception. The answer is that two IUIs in a cycle does slightly increase that chance—anywhere from 3 to 10 percent—but it also doubles the cost of sperm for that cycle.[15] Because it doubles the cost without doubling the chance of conceiving, we believe that one well-timed IUI is the best use of resources.

There are folks who still would like to pursue two IUIs in a cycle, especially when getting pregnant in a certain month could lead to longer parental leave, or when they aren't entirely sure of their ovulation window. When doing two IUIs a cycle, the first insemination is typically done twelve to twenty-four hours after the LH surge, and the second is performed twelve to twenty-four hours after the first.

Medicated Cycles

Fertility clinics often use medication to stimulate ovulation. The purpose of medication like letrozole and Clomid is to induce ovulation, produce extra eggs, and assist the luteal phase. These are the first-line interventions for heterosexual couples with infertility, and many LGBTQ+ people and solo folks get lumped into medicated IUI protocols. But the question is—do they actually work for us?

The answer is mixed. In one of the few larger retrospective cohort studies focusing on lesbian women pursuing IUI, researchers found that ovarian stimulation increased the live birth rate by about 0.5 percent, while increasing the risk of having multiples fourfold. The rate of twins and multiples in medicated cycles was 10.8 percent, compared with the rate of 2.4 percent in unmedicated cycles. Because of the significant increase in multiples without significant increase in live births, the study authors recommended not using ovulation stimulation for lesbians with regular ovulation under age forty-two. In addition to increasing the probability of multiples, ovulation-stimulating medication also increases the risk of ectopic pregnancy, ovarian hyperstimulation, and cycle side effects including mood difficulties and pain at ovulation.

There are folks for whom ovulation-stimulating medication may increase the chance of conception: people over about age forty, folks with PCOS or other anovulatory conditions, and people who meet the criteria for infertility.[16] If you are a person who is regularly ovulating with no infertility diagnosis under forty, there is not good evidence that ovulation-stimulating medication will improve your chances of a live birth.[17]

In doing the literature review for this book, what we came up against is that the data is primarily based on cisgender heterosexual women who are experiencing fertility challenges, and much of the data about solo and lesbian parents outcomes is sourced from fertility clinics using the same care protocols infertile cisgender women receive.[18] It's almost impossible to translate this data to LGBTQ+ people and solo parents not experiencing infertility to learn if doing a medicated cycle will increase your chance of getting pregnant. So our answer as midwives specializing in fertility care is that medication is sometimes an appropriate intervention that will increase your chance of conception. Unfortunately, it can also be an intervention that is used too early or inappropriately for solo parents and LGBTQ+ people that adds cost and risk to the conception process.[19]

Trigger Shots

Fertility clinics also use trigger shots of HCG (human chorionic gonadotropin, a hormone produced during pregnancy) to time IUIs. In a cycle using trigger shots, the person being inseminated goes to the fertility clinic a few times during their luteal phase to check hormone levels via blood tests and monitor egg follicle size via ultrasounds. When the egg reaches a certain size, the provider schedules a trigger shot to induce ovulation. This gives a four-hour window of when the IUI should be performed the next day. The evidence is mixed, but does suggest that trigger shots slightly increase the chance of conception for people without infertility.[20] Trigger shots do improve chances of conception for people experiencing infertility. For people who have a hard time tracking ovulation, trigger shots offer a clear time frame for when to perform an insemination.

We know that all this information about success rates can be stressful for people, especially for our clients over thirty-five. We just want to say that while it can be helpful to consider the data in your decision-making process, we also have clients in their forties who get pregnant after one or two IUIs. Fertility is dependent on many factors, and data is only one of many components to guide your decision-making.

> The temptation to change things up and constantly try to optimize conception was hard to resist. But my midwife, Kate, recommended that I do one method for three cycles (unmedicated with donor A). If you're not pregnant after three cycles, change up one or two factors. If you can switch to a new donor, do that, or switch from unmedicated to medicated, or both! You never know which factor might help you get pregnant, so it's good to change things up in a methodical manner. —Ellie Lobovits

IVF

In this section, we will demystify the most high-tech tool in the fertility tool kit: in vitro fertilization. Called IVF for short, this is the process of placing an embryo that was fertilized and grown for five days inside a lab into a person's uterus. IVF can be performed with your own eggs, a partner's eggs, or eggs from a donor that are extracted during the IVF cycle or previously purchased from a cryobank. When there are two people with uteruses and one is carrying the eggs of the other partner, the process is called co-IVF or reciprocal IVF. Fertilized embryos can also be implanted into a gestational surrogate to carry a pregnancy for another family.

IVF can be considered a treatment for people with infertility as well as a go-to conception method for LGBTQ+ folks, solo parents, and families using the services of a gestational surrogate. IVF also allows two partners with uteruses and eggs to share conception and pregnancy. Many factors go into people deciding to do IVF, all of which we will explore in this section.

What Happens During IVF?

IVF happens in two stages. Part one is stimulating egg production to have eggs retrieved for fertilization. There are different medication protocols used, but the most common according to Signey Olson, CNM, a midwife specializing in fertility and infertility care, is that the person whose eggs are being used will take birth control for two weeks, then begin stimulating medications and undergo very frequent ultrasound monitoring (usually every other day) of their ovaries until their eggs are mature. Along with ultrasounds, blood tests are done every other day to track hormone levels. Then a trigger shot is used to stimulate ovulation, and the egg retrieval procedure is performed by the doctor under sedation. For those purchasing eggs from an egg bank, the process of egg retrieval has already happened.

Once eggs are retrieved, doctors and lab technicians will create an embryo by adding one sperm cell to each egg. There's a huge range in the number of embryos that can be created through each IVF cycle, but often doctors can create multiple embryos from one IVF cycle. Success rates depend on the individual and the reason IVF is being utilized, and age is a big factor.

Once an embryo is created, it can either be transferred into the intended carrier five days later, or frozen to be used at a later time. After an embryo is transferred, the person typically takes progesterone and is monitored by ultrasound through the first trimester.

An IVF cycle can be completed over the course of one month or two. Co-IVF procedures are typically done over the course of two months. Once the eggs are retrieved, fertilized, and frozen, future children can be conceived without ovarian stimulation.

There is a dizzying array of decisions to make when utilizing IVF, such as different paths to take with medication stimulation regimens,

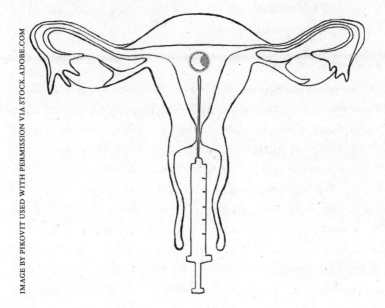

regular and mini-IVF cycles, intracytoplasmic sperm injection (ISCI) or traditional fertilization, and genetic screening with blood work or testing embryos with preimplantation genetic testing for aneuploidies (PGTA) to look for conditions that could be causing infertility or prevent the implanted pregnancy from growing. All these options add cost, and it really depends on your situation regarding which interventions may increase your chances of conception.

It is possible for an issue to arise at any point in the IVF process that stops the cycle from continuing. Medication to stimulate egg production doesn't always work or, sometimes, doesn't produce enough eggs. Fertilization may not be successful, or implantation of the embryo might not take. There is a small risk of experiencing complications from the IVF process, including mild to severe ovarian hyperstimulation, hemorrhage, and infection.

There's often an economics of sunk cost with IVF, and the idea that if you're spending the big bucks to make a baby, you should do every-thing possible to maximize your chances of conception can easily get the best of your budget. The challenge is that the tools and inter-ventions available may or may not do that. With all advanced fertility decision-making, start with the beginning: Is there infertility? Or do you just lack all of the components to make a baby? If there's infertil-ity, some of the interventions may be appropriate. Take some time to sit with your priorities in family formation as well. You can return to the exercises in chapter 1 to support you in this exploration.

Nature + Nurture: Reciprocal IVF

For some people in relationships where both members have eggs and a uterus, reciprocal IVF (RIVF) allows couples to create a child who is a product of both of their bodies. During RIVF, one partner donates eggs, they fertilize them with donor sperm in a lab to create embryos, and then the embryos are implanted into the other person's uterus. Although the process is very clinical and necessitates both partners taking medications and undergoing monitoring in a fertil-ity clinic, for some folks, this is their dream way of creating a child together.

When Maggie and I fell in love, we knew from the beginning that we wanted to have children together. When we were researching, we learned about reciprocal IVF and it became so exciting to us. I couldn't believe science made it possible for me to have a genetic child through the womb of my soulmate.

The embryo-making process was expensive and hard on my body, but I knew it was a drop in the bucket as far as the whole journey was concerned, so it was worth every dollar and every ounce of discomfort. We took out loans and justified them—people pay hundreds of thousands of dollars for their education, so why not make some monthly payments for a human who we will love unconditionally for the rest of our lives!

We got a lot of eggs, but unfortunately, after insemination in the petri dish, only five of them were viable. The doctor was so spooked by the rapid decline that he advised us to put three of them in Maggie's uterus that day. It's an uncommon practice that was fueled by fear. I was naive and spent two weeks scared that we would have triplets. Maggie was scared that because they weren't fully developed at the transfer, none of them would work—and unfortunately, she was right.

After she didn't get pregnant, we only had two more viable embryos (an XX and an XY), and one of the two was a very poor grade. We were pretty devastated after everything to have what felt like only one real chance. At this point, we tried for six months with my brother as a donor turkey-baster-style, and Maggie got pregnant twice but had two miscarriages. We had become really attached to the idea of having a baby with Maggie's egg and my brother's sperm, and Maggie convinced me to take out another loan and do an IVF cycle with her and my brother. Then we could have a bigger batch of embryos and go from there!

Unfortunately, we found out that my brother had a rare genetic issue that had caused the miscarriages, so we found a donor through a bank and used that sperm to create the embryos. We ended up with two embryos from her cycle (another XX and XY).

We decided we would risk twins and put in the XX from her batch and the XY from my batch, despite the fact that my XY embryo didn't seem to stand a chance according to the embryologist. At the first ultrasound there was one perfect little seed growing in her belly at last and we were over the moon. We decided to wait until the baby was born to find out who would be joining our family. There had been so much medical intervention at this point that we wanted there to be some degree of mystery and surprise.

We had a pretty strong feeling through the entire pregnancy that it would be the XX embryo from Maggie's batch because it was so perfect and what were the odds that the perfect embryo didn't work and the weak embryo did? We spent a lot of time thinking about girl names, and had a few ideas for boy names, but it felt silly to spend too much time thinking about it. I let go of the idea of being genetically related to the child and I was excited—I had always wanted a daughter anyway. Although this wasn't our original plan, and we had been so close to having my genetics involved, she would be mine no matter what.

When the baby came three weeks early on Maggie's birthday via emergency C-section, I heard a little cry and walked around the bloody curtain to meet my child and almost fainted when I saw a tiny profile that looked just like me with male parts. People don't quite understand how I could have been as shocked as I was considering that we put in two embryos, and one was from my body—but it just didn't even seem possible. We both fell madly in love with this beautiful baby that we had made together with so much blood, sweat, and tears. I literally can't imagine a better way for us to have created a family.

Ninety percent of the time people tell me how much our child looks like me; the 10 percent of the time that people say she looks like Maggie is everything to me. And yes, I did say "she," because at three years old our child let us know that she was supposed to be a girl. She was consistent and persistent and insistent, so I think in the end, we somehow got both of our embryos in one perfect human. —Joelle Schwartz

Affording IVF

The costs of an IVF cycle are staggering without insurance coverage—at the time of this writing, a single cycle averages $14,000 to $20,000, and an extra $8,000 to $15,000 if you need donor eggs. Due to the high costs, some people will travel to different clinics in the US or abroad for cheaper IVF.

There are a number of ways that people fund their fertility care needs, from switching jobs for insurance with infertility coverage (for example, at the time of this writing, Starbucks insurance covers IVF in full) to applying for grants, taking out fertility-specific loans, traveling for cheaper care, and negotiating with clinics for discounts.

Some people are able to access their health insurance to pay for some or all of the costs of fertility care, but many LGBTQ+ people and prospective solo parents run into the barrier of needing an infertility diagnosis to access treatment. It can be immensely helpful to have a provider advocate for you and challenge insurance coding issues that discriminate against LGBTQ+ and solo parents.

Whether you're able to work with insurance or you're paying out of pocket, remember that you can negotiate with your providers. Yes! According to River Nice, a financial planner specializing in working with LGBTQ+ people, a common misconception about the healthcare system is that prices are fixed, but things are often far more negotiable than you might assume. For example, River often reminds clients that IVF is negotiable at *every* step of the process, from the clinic you go to, to where meds are purchased, to seeking out coupons and consumer savings programs for discount medications. River recommends asking offices if there are medication samples available at their office, searching free prescription discounting servicers like GoodRx, and researching specific medicine manufacturers for consumer savings programs and coupons.

In the United States, CNY Fertility (based in Ithaca, New York) is known to offer low-cost IVF. People also travel to other countries for IVF procedures, where the cost of the procedure (even accounting for travel) is more affordable than IVF at most US clinics. A list of grants and other options for financial support around family building is available on page 284.

We want three kids. At least, we think we do. I am currently pregnant with baby number two and have an almost two-year-old at home. Whether we choose to have three kids, or stick with two, knowing that we wanted to have more than one kid played an important role in how we decided to build our family.

My wife had a hysterectomy due to fibroids so we knew that I would be the one carrying the babes. I was thirty-six years old at the time and had been working in reproductive health, fertility services, and birth work for fifteen years. Bottom line: I had seen the full fertility life cycle for many families. I knew that doing inseminations was less expensive, more intimate, and physically easier than IVF. I had also seen clients and friends go through multiple insemination cycles before they had success. Sometimes, they needed to switch from inseminations to IVF, thus bearing the brunt of both costs. I felt afraid of feeling the disappointment associated with unsuccessful IUI cycles.

We crunched the numbers. We averaged that it would take six insemination attempts for each pregnancy (times three pregnancies), with the understanding that it may get more difficult as I started to near forty. We were also banking on the hope that one IVF cycle would yield more than one viable embryo. We came up with a figure that was pretty comparable between eighteen IUIs and one IVF cycle. So, we decided to just forgo inseminations entirely.

None of the IVF services were covered by insurance. We were able to get some labs and an ultrasound with Kaiser. But everything else, including purchasing and shipping donor sperm, was paid for from our savings. It was a bit of a gamble. Thankfully, for us, it worked out as planned!
—Simone Lance

IVF Success Rates

We've been sold the idea that IVF = baby, but in fact the data suggests that IVF works best for people under thirty-five with unknown causes of infertility or no infertility issues.[21] With reciprocal IVF, the success rates are a bit higher and primarily based on the age of the egg being used.[22] With donor eggs, the age limit on donors contributes to higher success rates—48 to 51 percent.[23] The success rate with donor eggs and a gestational surrogate is 80 percent. The CDC has an IVF success rate calculator, which you can find at: www.cdc.gov /art/ivf-success-estimator/index.html.[24]

A NOTE ABOUT BMI

Some fertility clinics have a BMI cutoff for receiving treatment, typically between forty and forty-five. While it is true on a statistical level that folks in bigger bodies can take longer to get pregnant, size is not the only reason people have trouble conceiving. Weight loss is often touted as the answer, but we believe it's a poor substitute for helping folks develop health practices that increase their well-being and fertility long-term. Sudden weight loss and weight cycling have more negative impacts on fertility and, potentially, on people's mental health.

So, if you want to get pregnant in a bigger body, where do you start? We are such big fans of Jen McLellan's work at Plus Size Birth, and encourage everyone to read her guide on how to find a Health at Every Size (HAES) care provider for conception and birth, available on www.asdah.org.

What If the Plan Isn't Working?

Some people have challenges getting pregnant and will experience infertility. Our journeys are not always linear, and folks may switch plans, change sperm donors, add interventions like medication or IVF, or take a break from trying to address a health problem that could be contributing to infertility like fibroids or uncontrolled diabetes. One of the challenges with infertility journeys for LGBTQ+ people and solo parents is the expense, time, logistics, and decision-making that occur before we meet the heterosexual diagnostic criteria of infertility.

After months of planning and talking, we began this conception journey. Our simple proposal had been fleshed out into a strategic plan with lots of moving parts. Step by step, the pieces started coming together. Trips were arranged. An account at the local sperm bank was opened. A midwife to assist with inseminations was chosen. We even called our community together and had a fertility ceremony to mark the beginning of our "conscious conception." We were ready to start trying to conceive.

A few months of trying passed and we became more in tune with my body's fertile signs. A few more months passed and we decided to increase our chances with intrauterine inseminations (IUIs). At this stage, I received results of various fertility tests: all normal! We continued to trust that it was only a matter of time before we would see those two double lines on our pregnancy test.

After arranging our donor's second trip from Australia to the US to replenish our sperm supply, we were ready to begin again. Our first try with the new supply was a success! We were ecstatic!! After becoming such experts, or so it felt, in the world of "TTC," we had finally graduated to bona-fide parents-to-be. The first stage of our dream had come true—I was pregnant. Of course, we were aware how common miscarriage was, especially for first-time moms, but we felt like we had already gone through such trials to get our positive, so we really believed that this little one was here to stay.

We told our families, and then at eight weeks, we decided to share our good news with a slightly wider ring of close friends. It was beginning to feel real. Then at eight weeks and one day I started spotting. We decided to get an ultrasound to confirm that everything was okay. It was utterly devastating to be holding our breath, waiting to see that beacon of light on the screen displaying a heartbeat, and instead being told that the fetus hadn't been progressing. We were crushed.

It took several months to move through the grief of our loss. Yes, we tried to remind ourselves that at least 25 percent of all pregnancies end in miscarriage. We tried to see the silver lining that at least I had gotten pregnant…yes, it worked! But it was a very sad and dark time.

We found a fertility clinic that would support us with medicated cycles (using fertility meds to grow two or more eggs per cycle to increase our chances). We decided we would try four more times before considering other options, given our somewhat limited sperm supply and financial means. January came and went, negative. February…another negative. In April, we started considering switching to another local donor as well as beginning to research IVF as an option. With yet another negative that month, we knew it was time to make a change.

After quite a bit of soul searching, numerous heart-to-hearts, pro/con lists, talking to more experts and folks who have been through similar journeys, wishing on stars, rain dancing, tea-leaf readings, and everything else under the sun that you can do when you're making one of the hardest decisions imaginable, we decided to go forward with IVF. We want to keep our dream alive. We want to create a family. A larger family. We want to continue this path with our known donor. We had a dream, and we're giving it all we have to achieve it. —Lori

We know that the decision to invest in IVF can be a challenging one for many people growing their families. While IVF has a higher success rate than both ICI and IUI, the costs make it out of reach for many and a huge financial burden for most. For many people, the desire to have genetically related children is very strong, and individuals and families find many creative ways with grants, fundraisers, and loans to finance IVF.

———

Now that we've gone over the "big three" insemination options, let's talk a bit about the other things to think about after insemination— tips for managing the infamous two-week wait, and how to find the right care provider for you.

The Two-Week Wait: Managing Stress and Anxiety

The wait between insemination/IVF implantation and when you can accurately take a urine pregnancy test is about two weeks (for

IVF implantation this window is slightly shorter). For some people, these fourteen days can be somewhat agonizing, with the question of possible pregnancy feeling overwhelming and all-consuming. If you're someone having a hard time handling this two-week wait, you are not alone!

We love meditation, peer support, and professional support for navigating the stress of the two-week wait. In addition to the stress-relief techniques we talk about on page 86, we also want to highlight the following ideas to further support you through this time.

Distract Yourself

Sometimes it makes sense to resort to good ol' distraction tools when your mind is so occupied with an unanswerable question. This can be the right time to binge-watch that Netflix series you were vaguely interested in or take up learning the guitar. Channeling all that mental energy into something other than wondering if you, your partner, or your gestational carrier is pregnant can have a positive impact on your mental health.

Journaling

Journaling can be a helpful tool during the two-week wait. Some people keep a running journal of their thoughts/feelings about their or their gestational carrier's possible pregnancy that they eventually turn into a baby book for their child. It can be a positive and constructive way to get your feelings out and avoid getting into a possibly destructive mental loop of impatient anxiety.

Identify Your Anxiety and Question Your Thought Pattern

During the two-week wait, many people can get caught in a destructive thought cycle. Some people can get stuck counting the days or hours until they can take a pregnancy test, or start worrying about money or next steps if the cycle doesn't yield a successful pregnancy.

Try identifying which thoughts are causing you the most stress, and in a moment of calm, think of some way to interrupt that. For people overly focused on counting down until they can take a test, they may say to themselves: *Whatever will happen is already happening, whether I test or not.* You can also write this down on a piece of paper as a reminder.

Finding a Care Provider

If you're interested in pursuing IUI or IVF to conceive—or just want a checkup before starting ICI—you can make an appointment with a midwife, an ob-gyn, or a reproductive endocrinologist. All of these providers can offer a routine checkup and health screenings, though only midwives and doctors specializing in fertility care offer IUI. If you are working with a midwife or reproductive endocrinologist who specializes in fertility care, this is generally what you can expect when starting care and how long it can take before you try to conceive.

Midwife

A midwifery fertility intake is typically sixty to ninety minutes. In that time we:

- Review your health history.
- Discuss your menstrual cycle.
- Offer routine pre-conception health screening outlined by ACOG (the American College of Obstetricians and Gynecologists) for health conditions that can affect pregnancy and your ability to get pregnant, your blood type, and genetic screening.
- Draw basic labs and carrier screening if desired.
- Teach you how to track your cycle for ovulation and IUI timing.

- Review sperm options, and support you in choosing a sperm donor.
- Educate you on vitamins, foods, and lifestyle changes to support egg health and general fertility.
- Provide next steps for conceiving with at-home IUI.

Fertility Clinic

An intake at a fertility clinic is typically a few appointments, where they:

- Draw basic labs, including CBC, HbA1C, vitamin D, thyroid peroxidase (TPO), reverse T3, vitamin B_{12}, folate, STI, CMV, rubella, and blood type, as well as offering carrier screening.
- Do a vaginal ultrasound of the uterus to check for fibroids, uterine shape anomalies, endometriosis, polyps, follicles.
- Draw hormone labs, including estradiol, FSH, LH, and progesterone on day 3 of your cycle.
- Draw hormone labs seven days after ovulation.
- Possibly conduct an HSG and saline sonogram in the follicular phase to check your fallopian tubes.
- In a follow-up visit, discuss results and make a care plan.

Typically, the intake process can take a few weeks, so inseminations or IVF cycles might not start for two to three months after the first visit. According to Signey Olson, DNP, NP, CNM, who specializes in fertility care for LGBTQ+ families, one of the main things that holds up starting fertility treatment is getting insurance approval.

How Do You Decide Which Care Route to Choose?

Start by identifying your priorities in family formation (from chapter 1), then sit with the question of which of these options would make you feel most safe, comfortable, and secure. If having more information about your body through a fertility workup feels right before paying for sperm, then a fertility clinic is the right fit. For others, the personalized care experience with a midwife appeals more. Still others prefer to go about this process without the support of any medical providers.

Choosing a care provider is not just about finding the perfect match. Issues of accessibility, cost, and insurance coverage also play into decision-making. There are fertility clinics in most areas of the country, but there are not midwives doing IUI in every area, though many of us (your authors included) do virtual consultations to help guide people from afar.

Throughout this process, it's important, whenever possible, to find providers who are affirming to your individual situation, including family formation choices, sexuality, and gender identities, among other things. Friends, local family pride organizations, and the Queer Exchange or the Single Mom by Choice Facebook groups are often many people's first steps to finding a recommendation for an affirming fertility care provider.

Whatever you decide, nothing needs to be set in stone. Sometimes folks start with one model of care and then switch to a different model. This can be because of experience with providers, desire for less or more intervention, changing donors, or personal preference. There's no right or perfect way to do this process—but you do deserve to feel supported every step of the way.

———

Now that we've gotten clear on your *why* for parenting, discussed your options for where to get gametes, and talked about your fertility and insemination options, as well as choosing a care provider, let's revisit our decision-making tree for next steps:

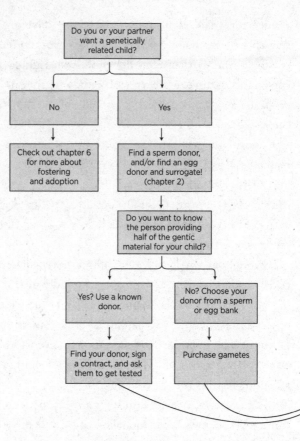

At this point in the process, many of our clients re-reflect on their priorities and their budget and start lining up the resources they need to start trying to conceive. This may involve purchasing eggs and reaching out to surrogacy agencies, asking people in your life for sperm, or setting up a pre-conception visit to check in about your health and start fertility care.

It's really exciting that you are at this point in your journey, and we hope that the path forward for your family-building process is

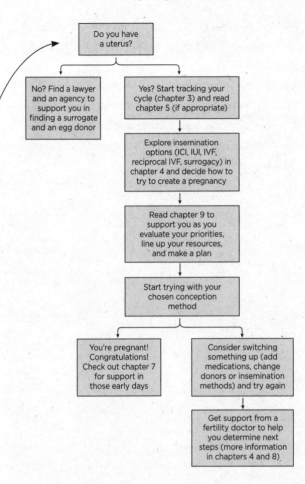

becoming increasingly clear. If you are trans or nonbinary and still wondering how all of this applies to you, head to chapter 5 to address your unique fertility needs.

The second half of this book is a choose-your-own-adventure of solo parent and LGBTQ+ family building. Some people want to know *everything* about this process, including what happens if this conception stuff works (see chapter 7 for information on early pregnancy), we well as what happens if it doesn't (in chapter 8 we discuss miscarriage and infertility). Others may not be sure that biological parenting is the right path for them and can learn more about fostering and adoption in chapter 6.

If you're feeling prepared and ready to make a plan and start trying to conceive, head over to chapter 9 to learn more about legal considerations for solo, LGBTQ+, and poly families, as well as community-sourced wisdom for navigating society (and our families) and tips for lining up more support.

CHAPTER 5

Trans People Have Babies, Too

> Since I was a young child, I've always known that I wanted to create life. I came out as a transgender male around the age of eighteen and I felt like I was a little forced into the idea of not having children. Once you start hormones, it seems as though society expects you to give up your chances of fertility. It wasn't until I was around age twenty-one that I started to see trans families in the media. I saw a community of people that were just like me! Men who knew that they were meant to create life. I felt inspired and empowered to live my dream. —Ezequiel Moore

If you or someone you love is trans, chances are you or they've received confusing, contradictory, or outright wrong information about transgender fertility. In this chapter, our goal is to synthesize the current information we have about trans fertility—drawn from both medical studies and our communities—to offer our beloved trans community the information they deserve about their options for family building and baby making.

As with most of transgender health, community knowledge and wisdom is far ahead of the medical industry. What we're seeing in community—and what is starting to catch up a little bit in medical research and healthcare—is that trans people who have utilized gender-affirming hormones are using their sperm, eggs, and uteruses to create pregnancies, grow babies, and have healthy births. There are still a lot of unknowns, but we can lay out the 2023 road map to understand your fertility and where to find more support for building a family.

In this chapter, we're going to walk you through what you need to know about how to use your sperm or eggs if you've used gender-affirming hormones, how to promote your fertility, how to create a pregnancy, and where to get help. We'll start with general information about transition and fertility, emotional considerations, and building a support team. For gamete-specific guidance, start reading on page 139 if you have sperm, or page 152 if you have eggs. We'll also talk about lactation induction on page 149, and pregnancy and chestfeeding beginning on page 157.

The bulk of this chapter pertains to folks who have used or wish to use hormonal and surgical gender transition tools before creating a pregnancy. We know that many people with lived trans experience do not pursue gender-affirming medical therapy, for many reasons, including inaccessibility. The recommendations for transfeminine and transmasculine people, as well as the community resources later in this chapter, will also be relevant to folks who have chosen not to pursue medical transition. There are a wide range of intersex conditions, and while this chapter does not cover the specific fertility needs of intersex people, we have worked to include guidance inclusive for many that will hopefully help lead you to the care you need.

We have spent many hours combing through the most relevant research about trans fertility and have spoken to transgender colleagues and community members regarding what information they most want and need about fertility. Neither of us have personal experience medically transitioning, and as midwives we both have more experience working with AFAB trans people than AMAB people. For this reason, this chapter has been edited by three trans colleagues: JB Brown, Emily DeMartino, and Camden Segal.

One last thing before we dive in: We know that fertility and parenthood can be a heavy topic for trans people. There's a lot of very gendered cultural baggage around reproduction and parenthood that may cause many trans folks to feel excluded from these conversations and the possibility of becoming parents. If this is you, we hope you can feel us holding your hand through the following pages, while also offering the expertise that we have gained through years of supporting the trans community through baby making and baby having. We wholeheartedly support you on your journey to parenthood, whichever path feels right to you.

A NOTE ON LANGUAGE

In this chapter, we will be using anatomical terms as well as community language. We use the terms *AMAB* (assigned male at birth) and *AFAB* (assigned female at birth) in order to note what reproductive organs people may have. We know language and community standards will continue to change, and what we're using in 2023 might not resonate in 2030, but we hope that the information presented in this chapter will help support trans and nonbinary people on their parenting journeys for years to come.

Does Medical Transition Cause Infertility?

Historically, when trans people have sought to access gender-affirming hormone therapy (GAHT), they have been told that they would become infertile. This is still present on many consent forms for hormones. The World Professional Association for Transgender Health (WPATH) recommends sperm or egg banking prior to initiating hormone therapy because of unknown effects of hormone therapy on fertility; however, without insurance coverage, these options are out of reach for many people. Research, insurance coverage, and funding to support transgender people's reproductive choices have been virtually nonexistent. So if sperm or egg banking was not accessible or chosen before starting GAHT, what does that mean for a person's future fertility?

Let's be clear: The only forms of medical transition that cause permanent infertility are puberty suppression followed immediately by gender-affirming hormones and/or the removal of the ovaries, uterus, testes, or penis without sperm or egg banking. Hormone therapy with testosterone or estrogen does decrease fertility while being used, but the effects may be reversible after pausing of hormones.

Trans children who have the opportunity to suppress puberty and then medically transition do not go through the Tanner stages of puberty, which means that their sperm or eggs do not mature under the effects of estrogen or testosterone—an essential physiological step to being able to create a pregnancy in the future. Going through the second and third Tanner puberty stages before initiating puberty suppression may allow for sperm to mature enough for later use, but this is less likely with eggs. There are experimental technologies that attempt to harvest testis and ovarian cells prior to initiating puberty blockers to preserve fertility, but these options are very expensive, experimental, invasive, and have yet to result in successful pregnancies.

We know that supporting transgender youth transition is lifesaving, so puberty suppression should never be withheld because of adults' concerns regarding future fertility. It's our hope that more parents and providers alike will proactively educate themselves to compassionately counsel transgender children on their future fertility in a way that fosters trust and reinforces support for the child's bodily autonomy and self-determination.

As we mentioned, removing organs, through orchiectomy (the

removal of testicles), oophorectomy (the removal of ovaries), or hysterectomy (the removal of the uterus), causes sterility. For people who experienced puberty before initiating these gender-affirming surgeries, sperm and egg banking can be used prior to surgery so their genetic material can be used in someone else's body. We discuss egg banking beginning on page 41.

In the following pages, we're going to discuss the research and fertility options available for trans people who have *not* used puberty suppression and have their testes, uteruses, and ovaries. If you have banked your sperm or eggs prior to starting gender-affirming hormone therapy, head to chapters 2 and 3 to learn about your conception options.

Hormone Therapy and Fertility

We're going to be talking about ceasing GAHT to use sperm or eggs/ uterus, because it offers most people the best chance of conceiving. This is a really big deal, and also not accessible to many trans people. If you are considering going off GAHT to create a pregnancy, we encourage you to take the time you need to process your feelings about this possibility, and think about whether or not this is truly an option for you.

Having a hormone experience that does not feel right inside your body, experiencing all the unknowns around the pre-conception process, experiencing changes in secondary sex characteristics that seem to change the essential you, and accessing healthcare spaces that are designed for cisgender people (which is most fertility/pregnancy spaces) can feel stressful and isolating. This can be an extremely mentally and emotionally taxing experience for many trans people and may affect your mental health profoundly. When you're considering ceasing hormone therapy for fertility, talk to your community as well as a trusted healthcare professional, and make a plan for who is going to support you.

Being off hormones was really difficult for me, way more than I thought. I expected to maybe feel a little dysphoric about my gender presentation. Early on, I worried a lot about what clothes I would wear. I prepared myself to not feel attractive or particularly masculine in what I was able to wear. However, clothes almost never became an issue and because of my pregnant body shape, most of my normal clothes fit for a while and then later, I could just wear one size larger of men's clothing. What I wasn't thinking about at all was my mental state pre-transition and the possibility of all of those feelings and emotions coming back, which they did. I struggled with social anxiety again and a lot of insecurity in general. I needed a lot of reassurance from friends and family about everything. —Sauce Leon

Sourcing Support in Community

So, how do you find spaces to be seen and celebrated in your transition to parenthood? Start with building your team! Talk to your friends who are parents. If you can, seek out a trans-affirming doula to help you navigate all the emotions around this huge life change as well as find your voice in care systems (many work virtually so you can access affirming care from anywhere). Connect online and through your local family pride organizations to other transgender parents. How do you want to parent? What support do you need in the life-changing transition into parenthood? Where can you pull in your community to hold and support you?

Many people have found online community support to be instrumental in their fertility and family creation journey. The Birthing and Breast or Chestfeeding Trans People and Allies group on Facebook is one of the largest places that exists for community support in navigating this time that trans people participate in. We are continually updating our website, www.babymakingforeverybody .com, with more current support group options for trans parents and parents-to-be.

HOW AND WHEN TO SEEK CARE

Some people who are coming off GAHT to use their sperm, eggs, and/or uterus will want information and interventions early to minimize time off hormones, while other people may want to postpone medical interventions and interactions with the healthcare system as much as possible.[1] Both approaches are great and reasonable, and the one you take will depend on many factors, including your own embodiment, your bodymind, your relationship to conception and parenthood, and past experiences and desires around clinical care.

Whatever approach is right for you, know that it's so important to have a care provider with whom you feel safe and understood, especially for experiences like conception, pregnancy, and birth. On page 127 we go into detail about how you can find affirming healthcare providers.

People with Sperm

Pregnancy is seen as a magical process of creation and is often seen as *the* mystical power women possess. Trans women are often left feeling excluded from this mystical womanhood because of our inability to carry a child and the difficulties we face helping to create one.

I mourn for not being able to carry my child myself, but that doesn't make them any less mine. That doesn't make being their mother any less magical. The true magic is not in the biological process of creating the baby, but is instead in the intense love and effort that goes into caring for a baby and child. My child knows who I am, more than I do myself at some points—I'm their mom! —Camden Segal

Before we jump into logistics, we want to acknowledge that some trans women and other AMAB trans people may feel grief about not being able to carry a pregnancy. This sadness can be exacerbated by homophobia, transphobia, and sexism, which lift up pregnancy as central to motherhood, invisibilizing other valid and powerful ways of becoming mothers and parents. If you are experiencing this grief or feeling unseen by heteronormative definitions of motherhood, we acknowledge this pain and loss. It's big, and spending so much time talking about sperm can feel demoralizing and out of touch with your lived experience.

We also know that there are so many valid ways to mother, to parent, and to bring children into this world. This book is about empowering our communities to become parents in whatever ways work—and while we are often confined by our anatomy, we are part of expansive queer and trans communities that are continually reimagining the bounds of motherhood, parenthood, and family.

Women, transfeminine, and nonbinary people who were assigned male at birth and want to use their genetic material can make a baby through intercourse, insemination with fresh sperm, or banking sperm to use in IUI or IVF procedures with a partner, friend, or surrogate. In this section, we're going to talk a lot about sperm. While much of the following information focuses on transfeminine people who are using gender-affirming hormones, more information about sperm health and improving sperm counts through lifestyle interventions can be found on page 90.

How Does the Body Produce Sperm?

Sperm is produced in the testicles, where germ cells develop into sperm under the influence of testosterone over the course of two to three months. This occurs more slowly when people take estrogen and androgen blockers. Although it is not impossible to create a pregnancy while on androgen blockers and estrogen, it is less likely. Trans people who produce sperm can improve their chances of creating a pregnancy by stopping androgen blockers and estrogen temporarily to increase sperm count.

Spermatogenesis, the creation of sperm cells, takes about ninety days. So, the first step in preparing for conception is to go off androgen blockers and estrogen for three months, then do a semen analysis to check sperm count (quantity) and motility (ability to travel) at the ninety-day mark. The results will inform your best next steps for creating a pregnancy with your genetic material.

Sperm can be tested with at-home testing companies, but you will get more accurate information from testing done in a lab. Laboratory semen analysis can be self-ordered and done at a sperm bank; at the time of this writing, it typically costs $150 to $250. Testing can also be ordered by a primary care provider or a fertility clinic; it may or may not be covered by insurance. It is also an option to check your sperm before going off GAHT as well as ninety days after to track the changes in sperm count and motility.

For an AMAB trans person, going off hormones is a really big deal, one that we recommend processing with a therapist, any trusted healthcare providers, as well as close friends and community. AMAB people considering going off hormones may feel dysphoria, or loss, or fear for their safety if their appearance changes enough to put them in danger simply existing in public. They may fear that thousands of dollars and hours of pain spent on hair removal will be reversed, or face changes to their skin, scent, body hair, and more.

It's a huge decision, and one that requires time and care to assess whether or not it makes sense for an individual.

If you decide that temporarily ceasing GAHT to use or bank your sperm is right for you, continuity of care with a trans-competent provider you trust, possibly your hormone prescriber, can provide safety through an uncertain and stressful time. A provider you know and trust is more likely to act as your advocate, which can look like calling ahead to sperm banks to screen for gender inclusivity on their forms, providing some fertility testing in their office to minimize interaction with new healthcare providers, or offering warm handoffs to fertility providers with guidance of how they can best care for you.

If your provider has not worked with a trans person ceasing hormones to use their sperm before, give them a copy of this book and recommend they consult with a local reproductive endocrinologist to fill in their knowledge gaps on how to best support you.

UNDERSTANDING ALL THE LONG SPERM WORDS

A typical sperm count (aka *normozoospermia*) is fifteen million to two hundred million sperm per milliliter of semen, or greater than thirty-nine million sperm per total ejaculate. Typical sperm motility is at least 40 percent of the sample being able to travel.[2] A low sperm count, defined as less than fifteen million per milliliter of semen, is called *oligospermia*. The complete absence of sperm is called *azoospermia*. The threshold for sperm motility "disorders," where fewer sperm are able to swim normally, is 32 percent. Low sperm motility is called *oligoasthenospermia*, and the absence of motility is called *asthenozoospermia*.

Does Hormone Therapy Decrease Sperm Count and Motility Permanently?

The research is conflicting.[3] There is research that suggests the effects of GAHT on sperm are temporary. A 2018 study of twenty-eight transgender women found that semen parameters were lower while on GAHT but were comparable to pre-GAHT levels after the cessation of estrogen therapy, which would lead us to infer that GAHT effects on sperm are not permanent.[4] Data from cisgender men who have testicular cancer and had their testosterone levels temporarily suppressed would suggest that the effects of androgen blockers are temporary, and that transfeminine people who stop GAHT to use their sperm would resume the fertility they had prior to initiating hormone therapy.[5]

However, we do see trans people with testes having challenges with sperm counts during and after the cessation of hormones. Estrogen therapy negatively impacts the Leydig cells in the testes that allow for sperm to mature, and some research suggests that prolonged estrogen exposure of the testes causes damage to these cells.[6] There hasn't been enough research on spermatogenesis following estrogen therapy to say definitively whether or not these changes are permanent.[7] A similar atrophying process is seen in the uterus and ovaries of trans people on testosterone, and these changes in AFAB people are now thought to be reversible.

Bear in mind that some AMAB trans people may have had unknown fertility challenges prior to GAHT. A well-done study on the sperm counts of 266 transwomen prior to initiating hormones found that transwomen and nonbinary AMAB people have lower-than-average sperm counts before starting hormone therapy.[8] This fertility challenge may exist for some trans women, although many will have normal sperm counts prior to initiating GAHT and after ceasing estrogen. Having normal semen parameters does not make anyone less trans.[9]

Can Anything Be Done About a Low Sperm Count?

The prospect of having a low sperm count may feel overwhelming while you're also navigating all the feelings around fertility, baby making, and stopping hormones, invisibility in your parenthood, and logistics with the uterus-haver, in addition to coping with all the unknowns of the pre-conception period and future fertility wishes. Luckily, there are lifestyle interventions and medications that can improve sperm counts and motility, as well as fertility procedures designed to assist people with lower sperm counts to make a baby.

If you are preparing to use your sperm and considering going off hormones, we suggest checking out the recommendations on page 137 and exploring these options so that your body and mind can get used to these lifestyle changes before temporarily ceasing androgen blockers and estrogen.

Additionally, many causes of low sperm count or motility can be treated in a fertility clinic setting. If, after ninety days off GAHT and initiating some lifestyle interventions, you discover that your sperm count is still under fifteen million or your motility is under 32 percent, we recommend meeting with a fertility specialist to evaluate for other causes of low sperm count including infections, medications, or structural differences. Your fertility specialist may be able to support you through medication or surgery to improve sperm count and increase chances of conception. Medications like Clomid and GnRH, which are also used to assist fertility in people with uteruses, can be taken to increase sperm counts.[10] You can learn more about infertility interventions on page 236.

Okay, Now I Know About Sperm. So How Do I Make a Baby?

What happens next depends on your sperm count, whether you would like to make a baby now or use your genetic material later, and also whether you have an available uterus and eggs through partnership, a friend, or a surrogate.

If You Want to Use Your Sperm Now

For a slightly below typical to typical sperm count, you can use the conception method of your choice outlined in chapter 4 with fresh sperm to create a pregnancy. If you're using intercourse or home insemination, you and your prospective co-parent or surrogate can track their cycle using the guide in chapter 3. Support both of your gamete health with nutrition and supplements, and inseminate or have intercourse once every forty-eight hours from the start of fertile cervical mucus through twenty-four hours post-LH-surge. You can do this on your own without help from a medical provider, or seek care from a fertility clinic for testing and medicated insemination cycles. If the person whose uterus will be carrying the pregnancy is close to forty or older, you might consider involving a fertility specialist early on to minimize your time off hormones.

For lower sperm counts, the type of fertility intervention is guided by where the sperm count is at. For folks with a sperm count between ten and fifteen million, IUI with medication for both the person with sperm and the person with the uterus is the first-line treatment. However, when a sperm count dips under ten million, IUI success rate per cycle declines.

With a sperm count between five and ten million, you can try IUI as a first intervention to conceive, but we would not recommend trying with IUI more than a few times. If a sperm count is under five million, IVF with intracytoplasmic sperm injection (ICSI, an IVF procedure where a single sperm is injected into an egg) will yield better results and minimize time off hormones. For very low sperm motility or if no sperm are found in an ejaculation, sperm can be extracted from the testicles and then fertilized with ICSI for IVF.

For trans people with a low sperm count who are in relationship with a person planning to carry the pregnancy, you may have the option to provide a fresh sperm sample to be used at the time of IUI for IVF. Fresh sperm does have a higher rate of conception than frozen sperm for IUI, so freshly washed sperm for IUI may boost your chances of creating a pregnancy. We talk about washing fresh sperm in preparation for IUI on page 33.

If You Want to Use Your Sperm Later

Some trans people will bank their sperm at a sperm bank to be used in fertility procedures or as part of fertility preservation prior to initiating GAHT or orchiectomy. Others will discover they want the option of using their sperm to create a pregnancy after initiating hormone therapy, and will choose to discontinue androgen blockers and estrogen at a time that's safe for them to bank their genetic material to use later. We talk in detail about sperm banking on page 81.

Alternatives to Using Your Own Sperm to Make a Baby

Many trans folks with testes decide that using their own sperm to create a pregnancy is not worth all the psychological stress and physical changes that would come with pausing GAHT. This is absolutely a valid decision, and you still have options.

People in this position most often look into finding a sperm donor if they have a partner, co-parent, or surrogate who will carry the baby. We talk in detail about finding sperm donors on page 30—everything from how to choose a donor to how many vials to buy—and then options for insemination in chapter 4.

DECISION TREE FOR TRANS PEOPLE
WITH SPERM

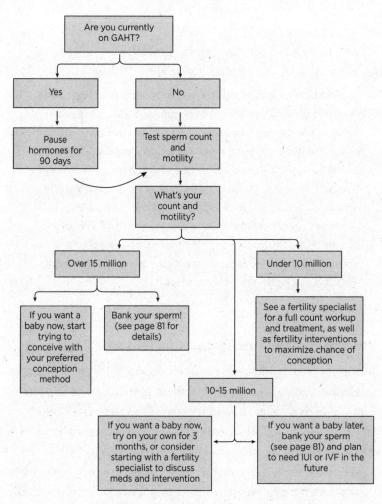

What If There's No Available Uterus?

For folks who are not planning to conceive with somebody who has a uterus, a surrogate is the most commonly available path to genetic parenthood. You can learn more about the social, medical, and legal aspects of gestational and traditional surrogacy in chapter 2. You can also learn about paths to non-genetic parenthood in chapter 6.

WHAT'S THE WORD ON UTERINE TRANSPLANTS

Uterine transplants are a new, experimental procedure and, as of this writing, have only been performed on cisgender women, though we hope that will change over the next few years. The first uterine transplant was performed in 2014; by the end of 2020 about a hundred had been performed around the world. The process of uterine transplant starts with two steps: egg retrieval and fertilization to prepare an embryo and transplanting a uterus into the intended carrier. About six months after the uterine transplant, IVF is performed. If a pregnancy is created it is considered high-risk, and the birth will be by cesarean.

Parenthood and the Postpartum Period

We imagine a world where parenthood and family building is genderless and expansive. Where there is room for each of us to define ourselves as parents in the ways that feel best for us. F*ck cis-heterosexism and all the pain it causes. You deserve to be a parent if that's what you want.

We also want to name that if you are making a baby with a part-ner, co-parent, or surrogate, whether or not that baby is biologically related to you, there can be stress and grief around not being seen as the child's parent, as well as feelings about not being able to carry a pregnancy. Additionally, trans people often need to educate their providers, family, friends, and well-wishers about intimate details of their child's conception in order to be known as a genetic parent, or will need to come out as trans again and again to be seen in parenthood as their full selves.

Transphobia is exhausting! When embarking on the journey of trans parenthood, here are some things we recommend:

- Line up your community to nurture you and see you in your journey to parenthood.
- Get the mental health support you deserve.
- Create ritual around bringing your child into your family.
- Surround yourself with images of other trans parents.
- Make a plan for postpartum (including infant feeding).

How to Induce Lactation: The Deets

All people with breasts can induce lactation—how cool is that? Trans people on feminizing GAHT can induce lactation to feed their baby at the breast. This can be a wonderful way to bond with your baby and feels very gender-affirming to many folks. The most effective protocol for inducing lactation in non-gestational parents is called the Newman-Goldfarb method.[11] It was originally designed for cis-het adoptive mothers, and has been used successfully with transgender mothers and other AMAB parents.[12]

If you're interested in inducing lactation to feed your baby, ask your provider to prescribe you a combined birth control pill with 2–3mg progesterone. Some trans people will just add a progesterone medication to their normal estrogen dosing. Then start taking a medication called domperidone six months before your baby is due, and longer if possible. Domperidone causes the body to increase prolactin, and birth control suppresses lactation—which mimics how breast tissue changes during pregnancy to prepare for lactation. The dosing of domperidone is 10mg, four times per day for one week. Then increase the dosage to 20mg, four times per day.

It's important to note that domperidone is not prescribed in the

United States, so people living in the US interested in using it will purchase it online from Canada, New Zealand, Mexico, and/or Australia. A US-based provider might be able to order domperidone to a Canadian pharmacy as well. There is some controversy over using domperidone in this way, because technically, this is off-label use. It has an FDA warning that it may cause safety concerns related to cardiac arrhythmias, cardiac arrest, and sudden death, but a well-done study showed that this data doesn't actually bear out.[13] The US equivalent to domperidone is Reglan, which we are not fans of because it can have greater adverse mental health effects.[14] We know that domperidone is used routinely in our communities for inducing lactation, but we still recommend discussing use with your doctor.

How do you order medication online? Start with friends or community members you know who have used domperidone to induce lactation. If you don't know anyone, you can try lactation Facebook groups and local lactation consultants (IBCLCs) to find out where they are ordering medication.

The person inducing lactation should continue taking estrogen, progesterone, and domperidone for six months. Six weeks before the baby is due or before the anticipated adoption date, they should stop the additional estrogen and progesterone and begin pumping eight times a day for ten to fifteen minutes while continuing domperidone through lactation. This mimics the hormonal shift following pregnancy that leads to lactation. You may add additional spironolactone to prevent androgenizing during the protocol.[15] You can also take lactation herbs like moringa (250mg a day) and fenugreek (1800mg three to four times a day).[16] Foods like oatmeal and nutritional yeast can support milk supply.[17] Don't pump or add lactation herbs before dropping off the additional estrogen and progesterone.

TIPS WHEN PUMPING

Put coconut oil on your nipples to avoid chafing. Pump for five to seven minutes on the low or medium setting, then massage, stroke, and shake the breasts to stimulate them, and pump for another five to seven minutes.

Trans people interested in lactating should discuss blood clot risk with their provider and possibly taking daily aspirin while on birth control. There is also a theoretical risk of prolactinomas (non-cancerous tumors on the pituitary gland that can be occasionally caused by GAHT). There is no convincing current evidence on this, but it could cause provider bias in not prescribing the necessary medications.

Another thing to note about using the Newman-Goldfarb method is that people with breasts, both trans and cis, using this method are unlikely to have a full enough supply to exclusively breastfeed. The amount of milk that you produce partly depends on your history of estrogen use—breast growth starts around three months after initiating estrogen, and it takes about two years for full breast development (Tanner stage three or four). Women are unlikely to get to Tanner stage five (full breast development) unless they had an orchiectomy before age twenty-two, so supplemental breast milk or formula may be necessary.

THE 411 ON SNS

With or without a milk supply or full milk supply, you can still feed at the nipple with the help of a supplemental nursing system. An SNS is a tool that uses a plastic bag holding milk or formula that connects to a small, long, flexible tube that can attach to a nipple or a finger. When the baby sucks at the breast or your finger, they pull the milk or formula through the SNS system. This is one way that people get the experience of chest- or breastfeeding without producing milk or while using supplemental milk or formula to feed their baby.

As a non-gestational parent, I induced lactation and co-nursed with my partner for thirteen months. I'm now continuing to bodyfeed our toddler and my partner has weaned. The journey has been full of sweetness, changes, challenges, and pumping! Open communication with my partner and allowing room for conflicting feelings have been necessary to make it through the more difficult times. I am also grateful to have worked with an IBCLC who was very experienced with inducing lactation and relactation. While I never made a "full supply" for our baby as an infant, I am a full contributor to our child's nutrition, well-being, and comfort. Inducing lactation is both mundane and miraculous—and it reminds me of the queer expansiveness of the body. My child likes to zerbert at my chest and laugh to themselves about it. Who knew chestfeeding could be so wonderful and weird?
—Lailye Weidman

People with Uteruses and Ovaries

Men, transmasculine, and nonbinary people who were assigned female at birth can use their bodies to create a pregnancy, grow a human, and give birth. Some transmasculine folks will use their eggs in another person's body with reciprocal IVF, and others will also use their body to chestfeed their baby, whether or not they are the gestational parent. In this section, we're going to specifically talk about people who have used testosterone and/or have had top surgery. Many transgender people do not use interventions like testosterone for many reasons including inaccessibility. If this is you, your fertility functions in the same ways discussed in chapters 3 and 4 of this book.

Taking testosterone suppresses menstruation and ovulation. When testosterone levels are continuously high, the cyclical hormone shifts in FSH, estrogen, LH, and progesterone that lead to ovulation and bleeding are less likely to occur, and reproductive organs begin to atrophy. While it isn't impossible to get pregnant while on testosterone, ovulation is erratic and hard to predict. That said, testosterone is *not* birth control, and because of unknown effects of testosterone on a growing fetus, it is recommended that you stop taking testosterone immediately if you do get pregnant while on T and want to continue the pregnancy.[18]

When a person on GAHT wants to use their eggs and uterus to get pregnant or harvest their eggs to be used inside another person's uterus to grow a baby, the first step is going off testosterone to resume menstruating. The process of stopping testosterone to resume bleeding can take anywhere from a few weeks to six months, depending on the person and testosterone levels/dosage. In the largest study of trans people using their bodies to create pregnancies, the average amount of time it took to start bleeding was four months.[19]

As we mentioned earlier in this chapter, we know that going off GAHT is a *huge* deal. If you're considering making this change, take time to think about how this may affect your mental and emotional well-being. Talking to a therapist can be helpful, as well as connecting with other transmasculine people who have chosen to go off GAHT to create a pregnancy.

Once a regular menstrual cycle has resumed, it indicates that ovulation is also occurring. With bleeding, fertility is assumed, and you can start trying to get pregnant with intercourse or insemination, or go to a fertility clinic to harvest your eggs to be used in another person's body now or in the future. You can read details about both options in chapter 4.

Both Marea and Ray have found in their fertility practices that ovulation often resumes before an effective luteal phase does. In other words, your body may begin producing healthy eggs before it is prepared to support a pregnancy. So, if you plan to carry the pregnancy yourself, bear in mind that it might take another month or two after menstruation begins before there is enough progesterone to achieve a pregnancy.

Does Testosterone Cause Infertility?

A growing body of research suggests that the effects of testosterone on fertility are temporary for the time you're using it and the months before menstruation resumes.[20] After that, people can expect to have the fertility capabilities that their body had before GAHT, plus the effects of age. The most compelling data is a 2019 study comparing the egg quality of cis women and trans men (who had used testosterone) after IVF egg harvesting; the researchers found no differences between the egg quality in the two groups.[21] We are of the belief that for people with uteruses who are stopping GAHT to conceive, we should assume fertility and well-being.

Hormonal Differences and Fertility: PCOS

One of the challenges that may have existed pre-GAHT that can pose difficulties to fertility is PCOS. Polycystic ovarian syndrome is a biological variation of sex involving elevated androgen and testosterone levels. PCOS is seen at higher rates in the trans and nonbinary communities than in the general population.[22] For some people with PCOS, the hormone picture can impact ovulation and increase other health issues that negatively affect fertility like high blood sugar.

For folks who were previously diagnosed with PCOS, who had

symptoms (such as facial hair or irregular menstrual cycles) prior to starting GAHT, or do not resume a regular twenty-one- to thirty-six-day menstrual cycle within six months after stopping T, we suggest meeting with a reproductive endocrinologist for evaluation to utilize medical interventions like medication to stimulate ovulation.

Lifestyle Interventions to Promote Egg Health

In our midwifery practices, we have found that the tools we use to help people resume their menstrual cycles after birth control or to regulate hormones with PCOS work well to help people resume a menstrual cycle more quickly after stopping testosterone.

Testosterone is processed in the liver, so using diet and supplements to improve liver filtration and increase blood flow to the ovaries can help your body clear out testosterone faster to resume menstruation. Here is a sample protocol that Ray uses with their clients who are stopping T to support them to resume a cycle faster.

Follow nutritional/movement recommendations in chapter 3 (page 83), plus:

- Prenatal vitamin with 400mcg methylated folate.
- Vitamin D: 3000 IU/day.
- Omega-3 DHEA: 1500 IU/day.
- Vitex: 80mg/day.
- CoQ10: 200mg/day.
- Alpha lipoic acid: 600mg.
- Eating seeds: Seeds are rich in omega-3 fatty acids and phytoestrogens, which help with cycle regulation. They are most supportive to regular cycling if eaten daily. Grind one tablespoon each of flax, pumpkin, sesame, and sunflower seeds and put them in a smoothie, on yogurt, on peanut butter toast, or on a salad every day.

- Castor oil packs: Take a large square of flannel, or an old T-shirt or towel, and soak in castor oil (usually about twenty minutes will get it fully soaked). Then you can either put it directly on your abdomen or wrap it in plastic wrap then put it on your stomach, and place a heating pad on top. Then lie back and watch a TV show or read a book. The soaked flannel can be stored in a plastic bag and reused for a week.

Trans Pregnancy[23]

This is not a pregnancy book; however, we want to SHOUT OUT LOUD EVERYWHERE THAT TRANS PEOPLE HAVE HEALTHY PREGNANCIES AND BIRTHS. In the research, the only complication seen around a transgender person's pregnancy is discrimination. Having a history of testosterone use, having had top surgery or other gender-affirming procedures, and outwardly expressing your gender identity full-time do not affect the health and well-being of your baby. What we find instead is that many queer people and trans people make very intentional decisions to parent and bring their kids into the world. So, f*ck discrimination.

In the research on trans pregnancies, we see that trans and nonbinary pregnant people use midwives and have home births at significantly higher rates than the general population.[24] In community spaces, we also see folks having planned C-sections. We encourage folks to seek care in the place where they feel most safe. Sometimes plans change and there's a lot we don't have control over, but starting with a plan and care team that makes you feel the most comfortable and secure will set you up for the best experience meeting your baby.

We believe that continuity of care, whether it be with a home-birth midwife, a hospital-based midwifery practice, a small hospital-based OB, or a family medicine practice, is the best protection against discrimination: When your provider gets to know you and your family, they are more likely to act as an advocate for your healthcare needs.

We also can't speak highly enough of doulas for all birthing people, and especially transmasculine and nonbinary birthing people. Having an advocate to help navigate systems and provide continuous support is crucial if you may be meeting new providers during your pregnancy and birth. We recommend checking out the Queer Doula Network at www.queerdoulanetwork.com.

Postpartum Considerations

At the time of this writing, there is no research on when to resume or start testosterone after having a baby. There are two aspects of postpartum bodies to consider when deciding on your timeline: perineal healing and lactation. Childbirth can cause injury to genital tissue as well as the perineum (the space between the front hole and the rectum). These injuries are repaired with sutures, which can take anywhere from a few weeks to a few months to heal.

Perineal tissue will heal faster and better under the influence of estrogen, because testosterone causes atrophy of the vaginal mucosa. That atrophy dries out tissue, slows healing, and decreases elasticity of the tissue, which can cause separation and bleeding. Because of this, we recommend waiting at least until perineal injuries are healed before starting testosterone in the postpartum, which for most people is six to eight weeks. For transmasculine people who birthed through cesarean section and did not have front hole tissue damage, it's possible to resume testosterone as early as four weeks after birth, as soon as the uterus has returned to its non-pregnant size.

Lactation Options for Transmasculine People

First: How does lactation work? The process of lactation starts in pregnancy. Glandular tissue is developed in the early months; colostrum, a thick sugary substance that feeds babies in their first few days of life, starts to be produced around twenty weeks. Once pregnancy hormones leave someone's system (around two to four days postpartum), this triggers the body to start producing human milk. Frequent stimulation by a baby sucking at the nipple or a pump expressing milk will tell the body how much milk to produce. If there is no stimulation, the milk supply will decrease and eventually stop.

Trevor MacDonald, a transgender parent and International Board Certified Lactation Consultant based in Canada, has been a leader in developing research and community resources for trans people who are using their bodies to feed their babies. In their 2016 study, Mac-Donald interviewed twenty-two trans pregnant people about lactation, chest care, and chestfeeding.[25] Nine of the participants had had top surgery prior to pregnancy. This is the primary data on which we base this section.

People Who Want to Feed Their Baby with Their Body and Have Had Top Surgery

Lactation after top surgery can look quite a bit like the experience of cis women who have breast reduction surgeries, in that you don't know how much milk you're going to produce until the milk comes in around day 3 postpartum. Setting yourself up prenatally with a lactation consultant can be very helpful, because this allows for early intervention in your home or in an office with a provider to learn how much milk your body is producing, and if / how much supplemental milk the baby needs to maintain a healthy weight.

Some pregnant people who have had top surgery develop glandular tissue that allows for lactation; others do not. How much glandular tissue was taken out during top surgery is the primary factor in the ability to make milk. People who have had double incisions with nipple grafts are the least likely to develop glandular tissue, and some will not develop any at all. In MacDonald's study the people who had keyhole procedures had the most glandular growth. Some of the glandular changes that could produce milk postpartum will be noticed in pregnancy through chest soreness. In the case of nipple grafts, it is important to determine whether the nipple has fully reconnected post-surgery and can express milk. If the nipple has not reconnected, the milk supply will need to be suppressed to prevent an infection in the milk ducts.

Typically, people who have had glandular tissue removed from their chest have a reduced milk supply, but can still enjoy the benefits of chestfeeding with some milk supplementation. Babies can get their extra milk needs through supplemental milk fed at the nipple with an SNS tube, finger-fed with an SNS tube, or fed with a bottle. When supplementation is needed, people use formula or donated human milk.

Better than science fiction is the trans magic of my chest—made more mine by top surgery and tattoos, but still always handled with care and distance. We had to get real acquainted. At the first lactation appointment before our kiddo even arrived, gloved hands helped me understand the map of asymmetrical scar tissue pooling in my armpits.

I went in wanting to know how to safely manage lactation postpartum post top (keyhole) surgery and left with the tools for a glimmer of possibility. We found two generous donors of human milk that would be the main source of our kiddo's food, but I wanted our kid to be as protected as possible and had read about the genius of human milk.

The plan was to give our baby colostrum and then be done—but our lactation consultant was a dream, fighting alongside us with so many types of tubing, tape, and tongue exercises for the baby.

So we got inventive—nipples became magic buttons, and the at-chest supplementor earned the name "juice box" for the satisfying sound it makes as the last drops of donor milk get sucked out. And I found it kind of magical, though never comfortable. Our donor milk had to be poured into this tiny plastic sack that hung like a necklace from a nylon cord around our necks. Each had a stopper and straw with a teeny tiny delicate tube that came out the bottom of the back and could be taped to my chest and guided by hand into our baby's mouth.

So feeding went something like this—each day we pre-made four to six juice boxes, as well as four to six regular bottles, focusing on juice box during the day and bottles at night when we couldn't open our eyes enough to struggle with the many steps. Warm juice box in bottle warmer, clip to its nylon and string it around your neck, tape the tube just so pointing out from the nipple. Slip a tiny tube into their mouth before they latch. Because of my top surgery, I also had to squeeze a sandwich out of my chest tissue to give the baby something to latch to. This process required three or four hands—but it was worth it. —Ty Marshall

CAN I RESUME T WHILE CHESTFEEDING?

We don't know a lot about taking testosterone while lactating, aside from that it will reduce milk supply. One case study from 2016 found that testosterone did not pass through human milk, which suggests it may be possible for trans people to resume testosterone and continue chestfeeding their babies. If you're weighing resuming hormone therapy and lactation wishes, we recommend talking with a lactation consultant and your hormone prescriber.

**People Who Do Not Want to Feed Their Baby with Their Body,
with or without Top Surgery**

Some trans birthing people do not wish to feed their baby with their body. Whether they involve personal preference, chest dysphoria, lifestyle, or plans around further medical transition, all reasons for not pursuing chestfeeding are valid!

For people who have carried a pregnancy and do not want to lactate, prepare to suppress milk supply postpartum, even if you've had top surgery. To suppress lactation, start taking allergy medications with pseudoephedrine (available at any drugstore) right after birth until the milk supply is gone. Minimize stimulation at the nipple or moving milk, and when milk comes in around day 2 to 4, wear a compressive garment on the chest with cold cabbage leaves or ice packs inside to reduce swelling. Sage tea can also help reduce milk supply—drink two to four cups a day.

There are medications available to people who give birth in the hospital that can decrease milk production depending on health status. Talk to your provider prenatally about this option to make a plan for milk suppression, and gather the items you need to keep yourself comfortable during this phase.

If you are considering parenthood as a trans person, you are not alone! There are so many other trans folks who are parents or are thinking about becoming parents. Whenever possible, we encourage you to start building community to support you through this intense but also beautiful process.

All people deserve to know their options around their fertility and reproduction. We deeply hope that this information becomes more commonplace in the trans and medical communities in coming years and that our beloved trans community members start receiving the care that they need and deserve. Trans people can and do become parents: wonderful, loving, and revolutionary ones.

CHAPTER 6

Fostering and Adoption: Raising Children Without Baby Making

Many solo parents and LGBTQ+ families are born through fostering and/or adoption. Some people know that they want to foster or adopt children from the start, because it has always felt aligned with their hopes, dreams, and values. Others may have started their journey trying to have a biological child, but then decide to change course to fostering and/or adoption after experiencing infertility or realizing that because of their biology it's not financially feasible to have a genetically related child. Others may already have a biologically related child and decide to continue to grow their family through fostering and/or adoption.

This is an incredibly common way to grow a family. In fact, one out of every twenty-five families in the US have an adopted child.[1] In this chapter, we explore fostering, fostering to adopt, and private adoption from legal, logistical, financial, and emotional perspectives. As we talk about the logistics of these pathways, we also need to center that fostering and adoption is about helping children in crisis— and this need may be different from hopeful parents' family-building wishes. For this reason and many more, fostering, fostering to adopt, and adoption each have their own important ethical issues to consider.

As midwives, we are not experts in fostering and adoption. We felt it was important to include this chapter because this is a book about family building, and fostering and adoption is one way that

LGBTQ+ and solo people become parents. So we've spoken to various experts about fostering and adoption, including social workers at departments of human services, adoption agencies, LGBTQ+ organizations, foster parents, and adult fostered and adopted children.

There are whole books written on this topic, and if this path resonates with you, we highly recommend that you check out www .childwelfare.gov to get a more complete picture of becoming a foster or adoptive parent. You'll also find a list of recommended reading and watching in the appendix on page 300. Our hope is that this chapter can be an introduction to this way of building family. After all, as LGBTQ+ and solo people we understand that it's not biology that defines a family—family is chosen, and based on shared love and commitment.

FOSTER CARE

Foster care is a temporary arrangement where adults—known as resource parents—provide care for a child or children whose parents are unable to care for them. Children needing resource parents range from newborns to teenagers, needing short-term placement to longer-term care. According to Randall Wilson, a social work service manager at the department of human services in Philadelphia who has worked in the child welfare system for the past twenty-five years, there are always more children who need foster homes than there are actual resource parents to provide that service. There are also a disproportionate number of LGBTQ+ youth in the foster care system. Up to 30 percent of foster youth identify as something other than "heterosexual," although sexual and gender identity is not tracked consistently enough to better understand how great the need for LGBTQ+-affirming homes really is. It is sometimes possible, depending on the agency, to request placements with LGBTQ+ youth.

As a foster parent, your role is to provide a loving, supportive, and stable home to children in the midst of crisis. Foster parents don't know how long they will be asked to provide this role—some children only need this support for a few weeks, while others may need it indefinitely. It's important to remember that the goal of the foster care system is always reunification with the birth family, but there are children in the foster care system whose birth parents' rights have already been terminated and have yet to find a long-term guardian or adoptive family.

How Does Foster Care Work?

The foster care system is a complex coordination among federal, state, and local organizations. Children may be removed from their home by child protective services, and then county social service agencies contracted by the department of human services place them with extended family members or other adults in their community (known as kinship homes), in resource homes with certified foster parents, or in group homes.

When the state decides a child is not safe in their home and removes them from their caregiver, the child is appointed a social worker who manages their case, as well as a child advocate who acts as the child's voice in court. The case manager's job is to work closely with the child, the child's resource parents, and the biological parents to support the needs of the child. As a resource parent, you may help facilitate supervised visitation with the birth parents, or be asked to bring the child to court hearings or appointments as specified by the child advocate.

Federal law mandates that there is a twenty-two-month period during which reunification can occur between a child and their family of origin. After twenty-two months, the law states that permanency (a long-term, safe home) needs to be achieved for this child. This is when foster parents have the opportunity to become long-term guardians or adoptive parents.

Regardless of a child's situation, ideally they receive thoughtful, trauma-informed care from their resource parents while their biological parents receive support from the state to make changes that will allow them to regain custody of their children. Unfortunately, reality often falls far short of this situation, where biological parents do not receive the support they need to recover from crisis. The foster system is deeply tied to the racism, classism, and xenophobia baked into the foundation of the United States. In an ideal world, all parents would receive the support they need to not become separated from their children in the first place.

How People Become Foster Parents

> My wife and I have cared for a number of children as foster parents, ultimately adopting our now-toddler. We started our fostering journey simply to be a safe place for kiddos to land, for as long as they needed, while supporting family reunification whenever possible. We parented kiddos for days, weeks, months, and years. We approached foster care not with the goal of parenting via adoption, but of parenting via foster care, whether it led to adoption or not.
> —Margaret Haviland

The first step in becoming a resource parent is choosing a foster family agency to work with. Foster care agencies are private organizations that screen prospective resource parents and facilitate placement and case management for children in need of foster homes. These agencies have different focuses and affiliations, including traditional, religious, focused on short- or suspected long-term placements, and others. In larger cities, there may be dozens of agencies to potentially work with, and in smaller areas there may be one or two.

Stephanie Hayes, the director of Philadelphia Family Pride, recommends choosing an agency that feels right for you: one that is close to your home and whose staff you like and feel comfortable with (you'll be spending a lot of time communicating with them!). Particularly for prospective LGBTQ+ resource parents, it's important to find agencies that are going to support your family, be allied with your specific situation, and not discriminate against you because of your sexual orientation or gender identity. We include more information for navigating discrimination in the foster system later in this chapter.

When searching for an agency, Randall Wilson recommends looking for an agency that is not only affirming of your identity but also has policies in place to back up that support if issues of discrimination come up. The Human Rights Campaign (HRC) provides LGBTQ+ inclusion training for fostering and adoption agencies, and a list of certified agencies that meet their inclusion criteria can be found on HRC's website.

The agency you register to work with will conduct local and federal background checks for child abuse concerns and a home evaluation to check for basic safety issues like working smoke detectors and no hazardous conditions like broken stairs or exposed radiant heaters. You will need to be able to furnish an independent room for a foster child (children over the age of five of different assigned sex need individual rooms). Once you've passed your background check and home inspection, the agency provides certification courses to become a resource parent, and once those are completed, you're ready to foster. You can foster as a renter and with roommates, but your roommate would also need to go through background checks.

There are no costs associated with registering or training to become a resource parent, and typically programs provide stipends for a child's living expenses, as well as healthcare costs for foster children. All resource parents should, though, be prepared that children may need additional services that require time and advocacy to schedule, as well as appointments and court hearings that require additional driving.

Once you've gone through the process of becoming a certified foster parent, you will work with a social worker to identify what placements you are open to. You can choose to foster a child or children on a short-term basis or to foster with an openness to adopt the child/children if that becomes necessary. Through the registration process, you will fill out paperwork from the agency with questions about what kind of child or children you would be open to caring for. For example, some resource parents specify that they are open to caring for children from ages zero to three, or are only open to receiving one child, or are open to fostering siblings who also need a placement. There is typically a greater need for resource homes that can take sibling groups.

Bear in mind that while an agency and social worker will try to honor your preferences, you may still get a call in the middle of the night regarding an emergency with a child that meets none of your descriptions. Experienced foster parents recommend being open to that. While it's perfectly normal to have hopes and dreams regarding what your family will look like, there are also children that need a safe place to go. As a foster parent, your job is to provide a safe home for children in crisis.

IS FOSTER PARENTING FOR ME?

Aren't sure whether or not you want to consider foster parenting? Here are some questions to help guide your decision-making process.

1. Does this information about becoming a resource parent resonate with you?

2. Would your friends, family, and community support you in this?

3. Would you be able to bring the same love, care, and commitment to a child who is in your care temporarily versus permanently?

4. Are you open to parenting children who have experienced trauma, have significant challenges, or may be grieving?

5. If you became a resource parent, how do you feel about the goal of reunification? How would you support yourself in saying goodbye to the child or children you care for?

As queer people, we already need to redefine what family looks like. We already need to question who we are in this society and what kind of parent we can be if we don't resonate with the idea of a "mom" or a "dad." So when my wife and I started exploring the possibility of fostering, and fostering to adopt, we were already familiar with the notion of challenging what family looks like. It required us not only to question the notion of family as biology but also to question the idea of family as permanency.

We have learned that family can change. For us, our family is our home, our space, and who is under our roof at any given moment. The constellation of who is in our family changes, but the love and connection among us stays constant. This perspective has allowed us to feel confident and grounded in the family that's being created in our home.

We've had to help our community and our extended family reorient to this type of family. This Christmas, our family is made up of two moms, a little boy, and a little girl. By summertime, it could be different. It could be one child, or it could be babies, or a sibling set. But it's still the Martinez family. —Monica Martinez, queer foster parent and CEO of Encompass Community Services (an organization supporting foster youth)

ADOPTION

Let's start with the basics: Adoption is a legal process through which you become the legal guardian of a child whom you didn't birth and in most cases aren't biologically related to. The process of adoption can apply to so many different types of relationships—from parents adopting an infant through an agency, to someone adopting their niece or nephew whose biological parents need that support, to a person adopting the child their partner gave birth to. Many people have preconceived ideas about adoption that have been informed by their family, culture, and religion, among other things. Our culture has convinced many of us that the definition of family is a group of people who are biologically related to one another—but this is not a capital-T truth. This is a cultural idea that we all have the opportunity to question and revise.

Chances are that as LGBTQ+ and prospective solo parents, you've already needed to unlearn many of the ideas that society spoon-fed you about how life should work. But many of us (ourselves included) have more work to do in unlearning biases that family is biologically determined. In this section, we will go through all the logistics relevant to growing your family through adoption—from how to register with adoption agencies to costs to the ethical considerations of building multi-ethnic and multi-racial families through adoption.

> ### FOSTERING AND/OR ADOPTION AS YOUR ONLY OPTION FOR FAMILY FORMATION
>
> Sometimes people start out wanting to conceive a child biologically, but because of infertility issues (or cost) need to abandon those plans and change course. If this is your situation, we *strongly* recommend processing your grief about not getting pregnant or creating a family biologically before moving forward with fostering or adoption. It will make a profound difference to you and to your future child(ren) that you are *choosing* to become their parent and are not carrying unprocessed grief around not being able to have a biological child. Finding a skilled therapist to assist you in this process is super supportive.

Foster to Adopt

On average, about half the children in the foster system become reunified with their birth parents.[2] But when reunification with a birth family is not possible, a child in the foster system may be permanently adopted by another family member or their resource parents. Some resource parents begin fostering through foster-to-adopt programs, which means that they only work with children whose parents' parental rights have been or are very likely to be terminated. There are many children in the foster care system whose birth parents' rights have already been terminated and are legally free to be adopted. The website www.adoptUSkids.com is the government's central resource for connecting hopeful adoptive parents with children needing adoptive homes.

Many people who are building families through adoption have a strong preference for adopting babies and young children without siblings, which means that older children and siblings are much less likely to find safe adoptive homes. There is also a need for safe homes for LGBTQ+ young people, which our communities are in a unique position to provide. Stephanie Hayes says that in her community, there are many older LGBTQ+ folks who have felt like they missed out on the whole parenthood thing because they didn't think it was a viable option for them, and many of them end up adopting teenagers (which catches them up with their parenting peers).

Entering the foster care system with the intention or desire to adopt a child is the most financially accessible way to build a family through adoption. It does not cost any money to register with the foster care system. The state provides some financial support if you are matched as a child's resource parent. There may be minimal fees during the adoption process.

Now, after having learned so much through this journey of fostering to adopt our two children, we feel uncomfortable with just about every part of it. When we started, our thinking was that neither of us had any real desire to be pregnant (and if we're really honest, mostly thought ew—haha!), that we think there are way too many people on the earth already, and that it didn't make sense for us to add any more. We figured that math added up to it making more sense for us to provide a home and a family to the many kids who needed it in the foster care system (according to their stats anyway). And we thought we'd do it "right"—we believe in open adoption and connection to first/birth family, we have a deeply queer understanding of family that isn't necessarily about blood or DNA, et cetera. So, we started the process—classes, home study, social workers—and then waited. And waited. And waited. I think nearly three years?

What we learned along the way is that, yes, there are a lot of kids in the system who need a home—but that's in large part because the system is broken and removes them from homes they know or supports foster parents instead of parents who are unhoused or struggling with addiction or mental health challenges. And that most kids in the system have a family, of course, but some (usually white, middle-class) Power-That-Be has decided that that family isn't equipped to raise them. And that broken systems and ridiculous bureaucracies abandon and demonize first families, leaving kids to languish in foster care, and, yes, can result in three years of an open foster family with no placement, even when there are kids who need somewhere to go.

We knew all this to some degree going in, but I don't think we fully understood the complexities or our complicity in this system until we were in it. It is a dizzying, confusing roller coaster of a thing to love your babies *and* feel guilty for raising them, to hope and pray they stay with you *and* agonize over their birth family's heartbreak, to know that your home might be the best and safest option for them right now *and* know that that might look different if their mom had gotten the support she needed, to live constantly in the present because you have no idea how long they will stay *and* try to create safety, stability, and a sense of family. It's one big "yes and" exercise and it's imperative to start from the position that foster care is trauma, adoption is trauma, *and* the families that are built out of them can also be incredibly beautiful.
—Rachel Devitt

Private Adoption

Unlike foster-to-adopt programs, private adoption agencies connect birth parents with prospective adoptive parents before or shortly after the birth of a child. In these cases, it is the birth parent(s) who choose the adoptive parents they want to raise their biological child. There are also some agencies that take care of placement entirely, in the event of a closed adoption (where the identity of the biological parents is undisclosed). Private adoption encompasses domestic private agencies, individual arrangements through lawyers, and international adoption through an agency. At the time of this writing, LGBTQ+ families are barred from international adoption in almost every country, though prospective solo parents who are queer can sometimes circumvent these restrictions by lying about their identity.

The private adoption industry was created for people desiring to adopt newborns. Almost everyone who registers with a private adoption agency is hoping to adopt a child right after birth. Occasionally, the birth parents of babies from six weeks to three months old decide to look for adoptive parents through adoption agencies, but it's very rare that older children become available for adoption through these agencies. Most older children who need families are involved in the foster system.

Open adoption is a form of adoption where birth parents participate in the process of placing the child with an adoptive family and may continue to have a relationship with the child and adoptive family.

Closed adoption is a form of adoption where birth parents have no direct contact with the adoptive family or child and may or may not be a part of choosing the family the child will be placed with.

International Adoption

International adoption is very complex—logistically and ethically—and that's why we decided to focus on domestic adoption for the purposes of this book. People who are interested in exploring international adoption must become well versed in the adoption laws particular to the child's country of origin, and these laws may or may not be compatible with the laws in the US. Having an experienced lawyer to guide this process is a must.

Prospective parents interested in international adoption must also spend time considering the implications of adopting a child from another part of the world who potentially has a different experience of race, ethnicity, religion, and ancestry as their adoptive parents. There have also, unfortunately, been significant issues with babies being adopted internationally whose biological parents did not desire an adoption plan.

Understanding the Private Adoption Process

To learn more about how private adoption works in the United States, we spoke with Mykhia N. Odom, LCSW, from the adoption agency Adoptions From The Heart. Mykhia works supporting both birth parents and hopeful adoptive families before, during, and after the adoption process.

The process of becoming adoptive parents starts with an extended application process, a series of screening interviews, and background checks. Once a family passes the initial interview process, prospective adoptive parents are required to complete classes on topics that may range from transracial adoption to open adoption, intersectionality, and infant care through the agency.

Adoption had always been in my mind as a possible way to grow my family. When I was forty-three and single, I realized that becoming a parent was something that I wasn't willing to let go by, and I also knew that I didn't want to go through pregnancy. I had seen some close friends go through the private adoption process and it just made sense to me. I approached it very practically and spiritually. It's like dating in a way—you put together your profile, you meet people, and it all comes with so much risk. I told myself that I would show up for every step of it. It was scary because I was doing it alone, but I got a lot of support from my friends who had also been through the adoption process. —Jess K.

The next step in adoption is home study and home visiting, which includes completing all the consent paperwork for adoption, reviewing references, and passing police clearances. Prospective parents are educated on positive adoption language and the agency's discipline policy, then a social worker comes to the home to see if it's a safe and adequate space for a child.

Once through the home study process, adoptive families meet with a social worker to determine their criteria for adoption—for example, whether or not they are open to adopting a child with a medical need, and their ideal age range for the child. The social worker assists adoptive families to create a profile that will be shown to birth parents. It typically takes four to eight months from initial application to being ready to adopt. Once your profile is available, you wait! Depending on your situation and openness to different needs, placements with a child can take a few months to a few years.

KEEPING IN TOUCH WITH YOUR ADOPTED CHILD'S BIOLOGICAL RELATIVES

Studies have shown that when possible, it's very important to maintain relationships with your child's biological relatives. This also includes *never* speaking negatively about a child's family of origin. In cases of adoption through the foster care system and open adoption (more on this soon), there are usually people in the child's life interested in maintaining contact with them as they grow, and this can create a rich community and extended family that supports a child's sense of belonging and identity formation. As part of maintaining your child's connection to their family of origin, many adoptees speak about the importance of not changing their birth name, both first and last name, when adoption takes place.

The Cost of Adoption

Most adoption agencies are fee for service, which means that you pay for each part of the adoption process along the way. Registering as a prospective parent involves multiple interviews and many different fees. Prospective parents can expect to pay a few thousand dollars initially to qualify and register with the adoption agency, then from $6,000 to $10,000 while trying to match with birth parents, and finally from $20,000 to $30,000 when they are matched with a child to cover placement and court fees. While costs may vary on an individual basis, according to a report from *Adoptive Families* magazine the average cost of adoption through a private agency in the US in 2023 is $43,000.

When an adoption plan comes up, such as if a baby meets criteria for a prospective family and they are chosen by a birth parent, they get a call from the agency that they are matched. Sometimes there's a meeting with the birth parent and adoptive parent before birth, but according to Mykhia, about 50 percent of placements are emergency placements following birth.

Disappointments and disruptions in the adoption process can be a part of some families' adoption journey. Sometimes birth parents will choose to parent after birth or during the revocation period (which is the time allotted by each state when a birth parent can revoke consent for releasing custody). Without disruptions, the termination of parenting rights and legal adoption can take up to eight months.

COMMUNICATING WITH FAMILY AND FRIENDS ABOUT YOUR ADOPTION PROCESS

Plans for adoption (through private agency or the foster system) can go awry. For this reason, people may opt not to discuss their plans too much with their friends and family until they are farther along in the adoption process. The benefits of this include that people may give you and your family more time and space without bombarding you constantly with questions or concerns. The drawbacks of this include that you may feel isolated through the potential ups and downs of your experience. We recommend choosing one or two close friends or family members who can support you but who won't distract you too much with their own emotions, opinions, and experiences about what you're going through.

Adoption—Not Just a Plan B

We've talked about the logistics of adoption, but we also want to talk about the emotional aspects of building families through adoption for children and parents. First off, the obvious—adopting children can provide kids with loving homes with parents who want them and choose them. Whether children come to be adopted through the foster system or private adoption agencies, it can be a blessing for them to receive stable care from parents who have the resources to offer them the love and care that they deserve.

In talking to many adoptive parents, we were struck by how pure and straightforward their love for their adopted children felt. Many parents who have biologically related children have to grapple with the idea, whether conscious or unconscious, that their child is somehow a reflection of them. Maybe they hope that the child will look like them or that they will carry on some sort of legacy from their genes or their ancestry. This idea can cloud people's ability to see their child as who they really are, without projection and attachment. When adopting, before starting the process, parents *already* need to question that assumption. This can be liberating, and can support parents to see the young people they are raising as their own individuals and help avoid potentially damaging projections.

Adoption is also very imperfect, ethically complex, and sometimes harmful. Adoption always starts with a loss for the child, and while every child experiences this differently, parents can harm their adoptive children by failing to navigate this loss for their child that led to the family the parents love and desire. When transracial adoptees are cut off from their community of origin, this trauma is amplified.

Additionally, one of the main reasons birth families choose adoption for their newborn is financial hardship. Meanwhile, families pay upward of $40,000 to adopt a newborn. If people had more equitable access to resources to parent, how many children would need adoption plans? Since adoption is about helping children in crisis, why are newborns considered desirable when older children are not? When considering adoption, also consider:

- How it would feel to support your child if their grief was directed at you or they rejected you as a parent?
- How does the financial inequity sit with you?
- Do you have community that is the same race and culture as your adoptive child for them to participate in, and the capability to consistently plug into their community of origin?

Navigating Racial and Ethnic Difference Through Cultural Competence

There are many ethical issues to consider when fostering and/or adopting children, especially for children whose racial background is different from that of their foster or adoptive parents. And for hopeful parents adopting children of a different racial and ethnic background, education on transracial parenting and racialized trauma is essential. Even if these children are deeply loved, they may feel underprepared to navigate the realities of race in our society. Or they may feel like there is a part of themselves that can never be understood by their adoptive parents. Parents adopting children with different racial backgrounds must do the work to unlearn racism within themselves, to educate themselves about their child's experience in the world, and to surround themselves with close friends and other adults who share in their child's experience of race.

I've gone through a huge range of feelings around adoption as a transracial adoptee. I've encountered a lot of parents who have a saviorism complex, and that's not healthy for a child. Adoption isn't about saving or rescuing kids—adoption is really complicated, and I'm very critical of it, especially international adoption, because it's a profit-making industry.

I'm adopted from South Korea into an all-white family that did not get any training on race or have much awareness at all. It was very much a color-blind love. They felt like because I was their child, racism wouldn't really affect me. I've done a lot of parent education over the years, and while I love my parents and my family and feel fortunate to have grown up like I did, I don't feel like they were at all prepared for what adopting a child from another country meant for me or for them. It wasn't until college that I connected with an adoptee community, and it was really formative for me as a young adult. Other adoptees supported me to process my own identity and make sense of who I am and where I come from.
—Katy Giombilini

A Very Brief History of Fostering and Adoption in LGBTQ+ Communities and How to Navigate Systemic Discrimination

Obviously, LGBTQ+ people have been parenting forever. But the right to be an out LGBTQ+ adoptive parent, at least in our current Western society, is relatively new. In 1978, New York became the first state not to reject adoption applicants solely because of "homosexuality." Then, in 1979, a gay couple in California became the first couple in the country to jointly adopt a child. However, various states continued blocking gay couples from adopting children all the way until 2015, when marriage equality became a federal law.[3]

To this day, there is discrimination against LGBTQ+ and solo families in the fostering and adoption systems. At the time of this writing, twelve states have laws that permit child welfare agencies to refuse placement to children and families, including LGBTQ+ people and same-sex couples, if doing so conflicts with their religious beliefs. Seventeen other states have no explicit protections against discrimination for people based on sexual orientation or gender identity.[4] There is an ongoing legal battle in the United States working to support the rights to adoption for both LGBTQ+ couples and single/unmarried prospective parents. A map showing the legal landscape for LGBTQ+ parents regarding fostering and adoption is available at www.lgbtmap.org/euality-maps/foster_and_adoption_laws.

Most states will license a solo parent to adopt, and most adoption agencies approve solo parents as well. Randall mentioned some bias toward single Black men looking to foster within departments of human services, and discrimination against cisgender men and trans people is a possibility.

Parenting Kids in Crisis

The purpose of fostering, fostering to adopt, and adoption is to help kids in crisis. Racism, systemic violence, and capitalism often create the crisis, and children in the foster and adoption systems may have experienced abuse, neglect, and profound trauma, even before they have the ability to speak.

As Laura Collins, a social worker who worked with a private foster agency and a former foster parent, put it: "There's no such thing as a child that comes into foster care or adoption that doesn't already have attachment wounds and trauma." Laura has found that resource parents who understand child development stages and the effects of trauma on kids are the most successful in fostering and adoption. Without an understanding of what trauma looks like in kids, resource parents may be more likely to interpret children's distress as a reaction to their own limitations as a parent.

WAYS TRAUMA CAN MANIFEST IN CHILDREN

- <u>Young children:</u> Irritability, startling easily, frequent tantrums, clinginess, activity level higher or lower than peers, repeating traumatic events over and over in dramatic play or conversation, developmental milestone delays.
- <u>School age:</u> Attention difficulty, being withdrawn, frequent sadness or scary feelings, difficulty transitioning from one activity to the next, fighting, change in school performance or getting in trouble, eating more or less than peers, wanting to be alone, frequent headaches or stomachaches without apparent cause, behavior common in younger children.
- <u>Teens:</u> Tired all the time, talking about trauma constantly or denying it happened, refusal to follow rules, nightmares, risky behavior, fighting, not wanting to spend time with peers, using alcohol and drugs, running away, getting in legal trouble.

HOW TO FOSTER SAFETY

- Identify trauma triggers.
- Be emotionally and physically available.
- Respond, don't react.
- Avoid physical punishment.
- Don't take behavior or a child's difficulties personally.
- Listen.
- Help the child learn tools to relax and regulate their nervous system.
- Be patient, consistent, and predictable.

- Allow children age-appropriate control.
- Be honest about expectations of your child and your relationship.
- Celebrate small victories.
- Focus on your own healing.
- Seek support.

It is vitally important that prospective adoptive or foster parents become well versed in the effects of trauma on child development and how parenting children with trauma is different from parenting a child who has experienced safety. The US Department of Health and Human Services provides more resources on how to care for children with trauma.

Attachment struggles are also a major factor in foster and adoptive families. The grief and loss process looks different for every child who has, for whatever reason, been separated from their biological family. Of course, children who haven't been fostered or adopted can also experience attachment wounds depending on their experiences of early life and whether or not they were separated from their parents and for how long. These experiences often manifest in different behaviors and emotions that can be challenging for some people to cope with. Although it's not necessarily possible to prepare for these potential challenges, it is very important to educate yourself as much as possible around child development and attachment trauma to have the skills your child needs you to have to support them.

Do Your Homework

Randall found that 40 percent of fostering is being loving and passionate and compassionate, and another 60 percent is doing your research. It's been his experience that resource parents who have created their own resource networks to address whatever the need may be are the most successful. It's a cliché, but you need a little more than love.

What does it mean to do your research when it comes to parenting traumatized kids? It often means figuring out how to access care for your foster child within the system while simultaneously building a network of other resources and foster parents to more quickly access support services like therapy or treatment for developmental delays. It's being willing to do more work when the systems are letting kids fall through the cracks.

———

We know many amazing LGBTQ+ and solo parent families who were formed through fostering and adoption. Although the logistics involved can be challenging, forming family in this way offers opportunities for growth and deep, lasting family ties. Throughout the course of human history there have always been situations where biological parents have needed other people to raise their birth children. Fostering and adoption are as old as time.

If you're interested in exploring this kind of family formation further, we recommend connecting with adults who have been fostered or adopted, as well as parents who chose fostering and adoption to learn from their experiences.

The ways you prepare to foster or adopt may look different, but they are no less part of the family-building journey than cycle tracking or choosing a donor is for other families. We encourage you to approach this process with the same joy, excitement, intention, and enthusiasm you would any other form of family building. The following exercise is meant to help you reflect on what you feel you need and want as you consider becoming a resource or adoptive parent. If you have a partner or partners you're planning on building your family with, we recommend each of you do this exercise individually as this can help create important conversations between the two (or more) of you.

EXPLORING FOSTERING AND ADOPTION

What excites me about building family through fostering or adoption is...

If I foster/adopt, I'm afraid...

Am I open to fostering/adopting a child with a medical or developmental need? Am I open to siblings? Why or why not?

How will I seek out resources to support myself and the child that I'm parenting?

If I foster/adopt, I will relate to their biological families of origin in these ways...

If the child I'm fostering/adopting is a different race/ethnicity than me or my partner, I will prepare myself and my extended communities to transracially parent in these ways....

CHAPTER 7

You're Pregnant! Now What?

You're pregnant!! Your partner's pregnant! Your surrogate's pregnant! Oh my gosh, *this is so exciting*! Of course, it's normal to have any range of emotions with a positive pregnancy test. Even with an intentional, planned conception, some people still feel shock, confusion, or overwhelmed. Intense joy and excitement are often present as well. We encourage you to welcome the roller coaster of emotions as you begin this amazing process of growing a new human being from scratch.

While this book is not intended as a comprehensive guide to pregnancy, it is our goal to support and empower you through the early stages of your family-building process. So, in this chapter, we will go through what we as midwives believe is most important to cover about early pregnancy. We explain common early-pregnancy symptoms and sensations as well as outline tips and tricks for feeling as healthy and supported as possible during this time of intense change. We talk about the medical choices relevant to the first trimester; discuss when, and with whom, to start prenatal care; explore the question of when to share your news with your loved ones; and talk a little bit about sex in pregnancy. Finally, we explore gender and pregnancy, drawing from the personal experiences of many trans and genderqueer people who have been pregnant before.

The bulk of this chapter is intended for people experiencing pregnancy themselves. Toward the end, however, we include a section with information and support meant specifically for people who are expecting children but aren't experiencing pregnancy themselves. Whether your partner is pregnant or you're expecting a baby through adoption or surrogacy, page 206 of this chapter honors your experience and offers some ideas to support you in the next steps of your parenthood journey.

This is a book about creating family and not specifically a pregnancy book. We wish we had three hundred extra pages to explore all the juicy, intense, and important aspects of pregnancy and birth for the LGBTQ+ community and solo parents, but for now we hope that the following information supports you during this phase of your epic journey into parenthood.

Exhaustion, Morning Sickness, and Hormones, Oh My!

Many people experience early pregnancy in a cloud—the tiny human in your uterus is constantly sucking nutrients from your body and simultaneously emitting unfamiliar and powerful hormones into your bloodstream. At the time of a positive urine pregnancy test, your baby has already begun growing their placenta, which implants itself into the walls of your uterus. As the placenta grows and connects into your bloodstream, it produces hormones that can make people feel tired, nauseous, and spacey.

Even though you probably don't look different on the outside, during the first trimester you grow an *entire human body*. A nervous system, skeletal system, and seventy-eight organs are all magically appearing inside your body while you lie on the couch and watch Netflix. It's an incredible accomplishment that should not be taken lightly. Given the enormity of your body's tasks, it's normal to feel exhausted. Or lazy. Like even getting up to go pee (for the millionth time) makes you want to cry. It's okay. Be gentle with yourself. Just because our society doesn't honor and support the work of gestating a human doesn't mean you have to believe it. We think what you're doing is the most important work in the world.

As midwives, we've supported thousands of people during this time in their lives and have learned some awesome tips and tricks in the process. While some of the following suggestions may sound simple, we know from experience that they'll help get you through the first trimester feeling at least mostly human.

Eat Every Two to Three Hours

This is *the* most effective trick we know for mitigating morning sickness. Eating regularly is a very important part of maintaining your blood sugar at a normal level and decreasing nausea. Even though many people don't feel like eating much besides crackers and applesauce during the first trimester, it's important to eat regularly (and even have a midnight or 3:00 a.m. snack) to give your body the calories it needs to regulate your blood sugar levels. If you can pair a protein with a carb, this is the best combo for maintaining blood sugar. Cheese and crackers, apples with peanut butter, a handful of walnuts, Greek yogurt, or a small bowl of beans are some of our favorite easy, protein-y snacks. If you're feeling too nauseous to eat most foods, try bone broth or adding a small amount of apple juice to your water that you can sip on and off during the times you feel like you can't keep any solid food down. While the juice doesn't have a ton of nutritional value, it will help keep your blood sugar stable throughout the day.

One more note about nutrition—don't worry about eating the healthiest diet in the first trimester. The baby is mostly drawing from the nutrients that have already been stored in your body from the foods you were eating *before* you got pregnant. How cool is that? So, if you're like Marea was during her first trimester and can only eat bananas and grilled cheese sandwiches or Ray with an all bread, almond, and berry diet, don't stress about it.

Take Regular Ten-Minute Naps

It may sound meager, but a quick nap really does help. If you can, lie down, put your feet up, and close your eyes for ten minutes, three times a day. If your workplace can't accommodate this, even closing your eyes for five minutes can make a big difference. Just remember to put a timer on your phone so you don't oversleep or miss any important meetings.

When Marea was pregnant, she felt out of it so much of the time. When she took the time to lie down and focus on her breathing, even for just three minutes, she felt more clearheaded and better able to engage with the people around her and whatever needed to get done.

Eat Some Ginger

Many people experience great benefits from consuming or even just chewing on ginger. People all over the world consume this cheap and safe remedy to decrease nausea. During pregnancy, you can drink ginger tea (add a little honey to make it extra delicious) or chew ginger candies (available at most health food stores) to get you through episodes of nausea. This isn't necessarily a magical fix, but for some people, it can really help take the edge off.

Peppermint Essential Oils for Morning Sickness

It may sound like a hippie remedy, but smelling peppermint essential oils does wonders to decrease morning sickness. You can carry a little bottle around with you and smell it periodically, and/or you can put some drops on your wrist or behind your ears. Some people enjoy drinking peppermint tea as well—just please don't ingest essential oils during pregnancy.

Acupuncture

We are fans of Chinese medicine during pregnancy, and have found acupuncture to be effective for many of our clients in managing nausea, exhaustion, and the normal aches and pains of pregnancy. Chinese medicine features a complex understanding of the body and how every system we have is connected, and it works especially well with hormonal balancing and support.[1] (Plus, you can take a nap during your appointment!)

Many cities in the US now have sliding-scale acupuncture places, and we highly recommend checking them out. Most acupuncture providers have working knowledge of supporting someone's hormones and fertility, although if you can find an acupuncturist who specializes in fertility and pregnancy care, even better.

A tool that comes from acupuncture that you can use anytime are sea bands! Sea bands are wristbands with a little plastic circle, designed to gently press on an acupressure point for nausea about an inch above the wrist crease. Ray noticed a difference instantly when they started wearing sea bands and found them essential for being able to get through a workday without puking.

To Say, or Not to Say?

Many people choose to keep the news of their pregnancy quiet for the first few months or so. This is because about 25 to 30 percent of pregnancies can end in miscarriage. The vast majority of miscarriages occur before twelve weeks, and in most cases, the fetus actually stops developing well before week twelve because of some unavoidable developmental abnormalities. The good news is that after you can see a heartbeat via ultrasound (around six to seven weeks of pregnancy), the rate of miscarriage drops to about 10 percent.[2] If you have a normal prenatal exam by ten weeks, the rate of miscarriage drops to 2 to 3 percent. Miscarriage is a big, heavy topic that we talk about in more detail in chapter 8.

When Marea got her first positive pregnancy test, she told her two closest friends and her parents right away. She knew, of course, the statistics—but she also had this feeling that that wasn't going to happen to her. And even if it did, miscarriage is a normal part of the fertility process that the people close to her deserved to know about. When she started bleeding just one day after her positive pregnancy test, she understood in a deeper way why some people choose to keep that news private. Not only did she need to grieve and process her own (albeit extremely early) pregnancy loss—she now had to tell her family and friends and hear *their* emotions about her pregnancy loss. And then, when she got pregnant again, she had to deal with some of their tentativeness in embracing the new pregnancy, because they were afraid of getting their hopes up again.

The potential of miscarriage is not the only reason people may choose to keep the news of pregnancy private. For some trans and gender-nonconforming people, pregnancy can invite new and undesired treatment from co-workers, family members, and acquaintances. For some, telling others about pregnancy means also disclosing that they are trans. Concerns about physical safety, as well as safeguarding a positive experience, may lead some people, both cis and trans, to disclose their pregnancy only to close friends and family members.

There is no right answer on when or whether to share the news of a pregnancy. We recommend telling only the people about your early pregnancy that you totally trust—and whose support you would welcome in the event of a miscarriage. Whatever your reason is for keeping this news close to your chest, we wholeheartedly support your decision. As with this whole process, do what feels right, and try your best not to feel bad about whichever path you choose.

I decided not to announce my pregnancy on the internet because I didn't want the experience of being misgendered and called mom online. I told my family I was pregnant around sixteen weeks with a "queer pregnancy primer" email, explaining how I conceived, that the donor was not a dad, our parenting terms and how we're navigating gender with our baby. It felt good to set our boundaries from the get-go, but more challenging than I expected to have to reinforce these boundaries over and over. —Til

EARLY-PREGNANCY ANXIETY

There are so many aspects of the reproductive experience that have the potential to cause anxiety. Many people, particularly those who have experienced pregnancy loss, feel anxiety or fear surrounding their baby's well-being in early pregnancy. Ray, who experienced two miscarriages, was immensely anxious in the first few weeks of pregnancy every time their nausea would subside. It's hard not to feel fear when you have experienced loss. And even if you have never experienced pregnancy loss, it's common to feel some level of concern in the first trimester, before you can feel the baby move or notice tangible physical changes as your body grows. If you, like millions of other newly pregnant people, experience some level of anxiety during your early pregnancy, the tools presented on page 86 can help. In addition, here are a few extra ones specific to early pregnancy.

Get Good Care: First of all, it's very important to have a care provider (or three) whom you trust to help you navigate this time. A midwife can reassure you or come over to your home to listen to the baby's heartbeat with a

Doppler or order an ultrasound. A therapist could help give you personalized tools to navigate your anxiety as well as hold the bigger picture of your mental health needs. A doula can offer emotional support tools during this time as well. The bottom line is that having care you trust goes a long way during the sometimes especially stressful time of early pregnancy.

Use Affirmations: Studies have shown that stating positive affirmations actually has a tangible positive impact on mental health and well-being.[3] When you state a positive affirmation, your brain and body respond as if what you are saying is happening in the external world. For this reason, positive affirmations are a powerful tool in reducing early-pregnancy anxiety (and anxiety in general). Repeating to yourself statements like "My baby is healthy and thriving" or "My body is the right home for my growing baby" can be powerful in moments of anxiety. Come up with your own affirmations, write them on sticky notes, and put them all over your house. Ray, who has a block around even using the word *affirmations*, finds that gratitude lists are helpful and provide similar redirection.

Exercise: Exercise is deeply supportive of our mental health. It reduces anxiety and depression, lifts negative moods, boosts self-esteem, and improves cognitive function.[4] Early pregnancy isn't the right time to train for a marathon (especially if you've never done it before), but it is a great time to go on long walks, do prenatal yoga, and take on some light strength training. It's safe to continue any exercises you were doing before pregnancy—just listen to your body, stay hydrated, and don't push yourself too hard.

Distract Yourself: Sometimes, you just have to take your mind off it. Give yourself permission to binge-watch that Netflix series you were vaguely interested in or take up learning the guitar. Sometimes you're just too sick and exhausted to do anything except play endless solitaire on your phone—and that's okay. Channeling all that mental energy into something other than constantly wondering if you're still pregnant can have a positive impact on your mental health.

Once you're pregnant, it can feel like the wheels of the medical-industrial complex are set into irrevocable motion. You have to make a lot of decisions about everything from your care provider to what tests and information you'd like about your fetus—and you have to make them fast, at a time when you're likely exhausted, nauseous, and anxious. Knowing what's on deck and giving yourself a chance to reflect at a time that feels less stressful for you can result in a more positive, supportive experience.

As midwives, we are huge proponents of bodily autonomy, and we want to remind you that you—*yes, you!*—are in charge of your medical care and *everything* that happens to your body. Many of us are conditioned to forget this fact when we go to the doctor, and it can sometimes be an uphill battle to unlearn this conditioning. Consider this your reminder that you don't *have* to do anything that you don't want to do. It is your healthcare provider's job to provide you with options and the information you need to make an informed decision about your options.

When Should I Start Getting Prenatal Care?

Most people begin getting prenatal care sometime during the first trimester. Some people opt to start prenatal care as early as the sixth week of pregnancy (two weeks after your positive pregnancy test), because this is when we can start seeing the tiny, beating heart inside the uterus via ultrasound technology. Others may wait until week twelve when we can hear the heartbeat with a handheld Doppler. If you're experiencing early-pregnancy anxiety, have other health issues, or are simply wanting to connect with your healthcare provider to receive some care, you may opt to start seeing them sooner rather than later.

At your first prenatal visit, your provider will draw labs that are standard in early pregnancy and will most likely offer an ultrasound to confirm that you have a viable, intrauterine pregnancy. Prenatal visits usually occur once a month in the beginning of pregnancy, then get more frequent as the pregnancy progresses. People with preexisting health conditions or conditions that develop in pregnancy may have more frequent visits.

What's the Difference Between an Obstetrician and a Midwife?

The main difference between obstetricians (OBs) and midwives is that an obstetrician is a trained surgeon and an expert in complicated pregnancies and births, and midwives are experts in normal, low-risk pregnancies and births. Low-risk means not having preexisting conditions like hypertension or a clotting disorder, or developing a prenatal condition like preeclampsia that can affect the health and well-being of you or the baby during pregnancy, birth, or postpartum. Eighty-five percent of pregnant people are considered to be low-risk, and midwives work with doctors to transition care if a health issue develops.

In the United States, there are two types of midwives: those trained outside hospitals (licensed midwives or certified professional midwives) and those trained inside (certified nurse midwives). Out-of-hospital midwives are usually licensed by the medical board in their particular state, and hospital-based midwives are licensed by the Board of Registered Nurses. At the time of this writing, out-of-hospital midwifery is either unregulated or illegal in sixteen states.[5]

Though there is little difference in the services that in-hospital and out-of-hospital midwives or obstetricians offer, a key difference between them is the time that they can spend with you. Most out-of-hospital midwives offer prenatal appointments that last about one hour, whereas hospital-based midwife visits can range from ten to forty minutes, and obstetrician appointments typically range from five to fifteen minutes. Birth centers, which may be staffed by CPMs or CNMs depending on state laws, may have prenatal appointments ranging from fifteen to sixty minutes. There is also often a difference in the style of care and the tools and interventions available to care for you during birth in different settings.

And, okay, we're biased. As two out-of-hospital-based midwives we *strongly* believe in the power of midwifery care in every care setting. It can make such a difference to have a compassionate, skilled provider, based in your own community, who can hold your hand and support you through your entire pregnancy, birth, and postpartum period. But we also acknowledge that not everyone has access to midwives. There are barriers around cost, bias, insurance, and health status that can get in the way of people finding or working with midwives.

Regardless of which path you choose, if you have options with your insurance company, we recommend meeting with a couple of different providers to get a sense of their style of care before committing. People feel safe with different providers, whether around criteria of race, sex, gender, experience, or personality type. And you deserve to feel safe during your pregnancy care. We offer concrete advice for finding the right provider for you on page 127.

I had four IUIs, two at home and two at a fertility clinic. The home experience was lovely—I learned so much about listening to my body's cues and what I needed to go into the process with purpose. Because I was going into parenthood without a partner it was important to me that I felt connected and cared for by the people involved. Moving to the clinic was the exact opposite—I never knew what was happening, I felt like the doctors weren't seeing me as a whole person, and the one IUI I had that was performed by a doctor was the most uncomfortable as unnecessary equipment was used. Having come from such a tender home experience made the clinic experience all the worse, but I feel lucky to have had it because it opened my eyes to holistic care and ultimately my choice to go with midwives at home rather than the hospital. —Meredith Nutting

Early Tests and Ultrasounds

Lab Tests

At your first appointment, your midwife or doctor will likely discuss with you your options for lab tests and ultrasounds. Initial labs include tests that check your blood type, your iron and vitamin D levels, your STI status, your immunity to rubella, your HIV status, and others. You'll also have the option to do genetic screening or testing. This, as with everything, is a personal choice that we recommend putting some thought into.

Some people approach genetic screening or testing with the sentiment that they want to know whatever information they can about the person growing inside them. Others feel like they don't want to impact their budding relationship with their little one with these tests. Some might choose to terminate the pregnancy based on the results of the test—others wouldn't dream of it. You'll be able to discuss your risk factors and the pros and cons of testing with your provider, but it can be helpful to think about your feelings about genetic screening and discuss with a partner or friend before your initial appointment.

Early Ultrasounds

As mentioned earlier, we are able to see the little person's beating heart at around six weeks of pregnancy. The medical industry insists that ultrasound technology is safe for tiny babies, and we mostly agree. There is good evidence that two to three ultrasounds over the course of a pregnancy improves outcomes for babies. However, ultrasound technology heats tissue, and since we don't yet understand the effects of this, there is general consensus in the research to minimize ultrasound exposure to necessary exams during pregnancy.[6] Follow your gut when it comes to making your decision about your early ultrasound.

Before Marea got pregnant, her plan was to only do one ultrasound at twenty weeks. She thought that she didn't want to expose the baby to ultrasound technology at such a tiny, tender age. And then, after her chemical pregnancy, she was terrified that it would happen again. She couldn't feel her uterus growing (it stays behind the pubic bone until about ten weeks) and was way more anxious than she thought she would be. So she got an early ultrasound. Seeing her little baby wiggle in there calmed her anxiety immensely. It was a great decision, even though it was the opposite of what she had originally planned.

So whether it's about the early ultrasound, genetic testing, or choosing between a midwife and an OB, let yourself change your mind. There is no right path in life, in pregnancy, or in parenthood. We just recommend understanding your options and choosing your path with intention.

Finding Out Your Baby's Sex Before Birth

Some people feel compelled to find out their baby's sex prenatally, while others do not. While we don't believe that there is one right answer, we do encourage you to think beforehand about why you want this information and how it might inform your own experience of pregnancy and that of the people around you.

If you do decide to find out your baby's sex before birth, there are two ways to do this. The first is via ultrasound at about twenty weeks of pregnancy (this is mostly accurate, but occasionally, sonographers do make mistakes). The other option is through noninvasive prenatal testing, or NIPT, where your provider will draw your blood and then the lab can determine the baby's sex via fetal DNA found in your bloodstream. This method is almost 100 percent accurate as well, unless someone is carrying twins, in which case it may only analyze the DNA of one of the babies.

Although many people in our society find it compelling to find out the sex of their babies before their arrival (and assume that sex equals gender), this process does encourage an intense gendered experience for the fetus even before they are born. It's been well documented that male babies are more frequently referred to as "strong" while female babies are more frequently referred to as "sweet" or "beautiful."[7] Many people, especially in the queer community, try to shield their babies from this gendered experience as much as possible, maybe even deciding to use "they" pronouns or all pronouns for their children until their child can choose their gender for themselves.

> We decided to find out our baby's sex before birth because I knew that I would have tons of feelings if we had a male child. I wanted to give myself time to process that information so that when my baby was born I could love

him like he deserved, and not be clouded by disappointment informed by my trauma around living in a sexist and patriarchal society.—Hannah

My partner and I knew we would not find out the sex from the very beginning. We wanted the longest possible time to build a relationship with our baby without having to navigate society's BS about gender and babies. —Til

Sex and Pregnancy

Sex during pregnancy is safe,[8] and many people experience pregnancy as an extra-sensual and connected time within their own bodies and sometimes, if applicable, with their partners. Sex can even support a healthy pregnancy—orgasm causes contractions that can strengthen the uterus, and they increase blood flow to the uterus and placenta (and therefore, to the baby). There are also people whose sex drive decreases during pregnancy, which is a less-talked-about but also common experience.

Generally, all types of consensual sex are safe during pregnancy, including anal or oral sex, unless you're experiencing certain pregnancy complications. If you're having sex with multiple partners while pregnant, we strongly recommend being extra cognizant of protecting yourself from sexually transmitted infections, some of which have the potential to negatively affect the baby.

With rougher sex and kink, it's important to take extra precautions to avoid abdominal trauma during pregnancy. Hormonal and uterine changes in pregnancy will change your pelvic floor, and that can make people more susceptible to tweaking a muscle or experiencing a pelvic floor or pubic symphysis injury. With sex, kink, and basically everything else in pregnancy, start slow, listen to your body, and be open to your desires and abilities changing as your body changes.

Gender and Pregnancy

Getting aggressively gendered as a "mommy" while I was out in the world meant I really valued coming home to my queer/trans bubble, where my partner and my closest friends all saw me and my gender and didn't change how they interacted with me just because I was growing a human. Also helpful: having my partner and friends come with me and advocate for me to be gendered correctly and access consent-oriented care at our OB's office, at couples' yoga, and with our midwives. —Mika

Pregnancy is an inherently human experience that doesn't have a gender, and a person's gender identity is not necessarily connected to their desire to carry and birth a child. Unfortunately, there are many people in our society who are attached to the notion that pregnancy is a feminine, "womanly" thing to do. These cultural ideas can create a challenging experience of gender dysphoria for genderqueer and trans people who are pregnant. In this section, we include excerpts from genderqueer and trans people who have been pregnant and were willing to share their experiences with us. We also share some community-sourced resources for support if you are experiencing challenging gender feels during your pregnancy.

While everybody's experience of pregnancy is unique to them, we know that there are also themes to what many LGBTQ+ and solo parents experience around changes in their bodies, hearts, and gender expressions.

There are advantages to being a pregnant man and there are challenges. Privacy is the big thing that comes to mind, and it cut both ways. No one felt entitled to touch me without permission. No one came up to me in the grocery store to feel my belly. But I had to reveal quite a bit about myself if I wanted to share the happiness, excitement, or discomfort of pregnancy with them. Everything felt too fragile. I've never had very thick skin and I didn't have the strength to shelter my growing child from hurtful words.

Curiosity is a powerful impulse and even the most well-intentioned people can have trouble curbing it. If I didn't say anything I might be asked:

"Are you adopting?"

Oh, that's actually personal.

"Are you using a surrogate?"

Yeah, like I said…

If I just said, "I'm pregnant," I got:

"How far along is your wife?"

Oh, I have a boyfriend.

"…"

And if I spelled the whole thing out I sometimes got:

"Are you transitioning back?"

or

"I thought you had, ya know, other surgery…"

or

"I'm not sure if I should ask this but how did the baby get inside?"

I try not to think about those moments much, both because they weren't meant to be hurtful and more important because they are irrelevant. I was busy being hopeful, tired, scared, nauseous, full of wonder, versatile, protective, gifted, and just inherently human.

—Eli Wise

Genderqueer and trans people have been experiencing pregnancy forever, and lucky for us, we are at a point in human history when more and more genderqueer and trans people are getting pregnant, having babies, and being open about their experiences. For those of you who are genderqueer and/or trans and planning to get pregnant, here is some community-sourced advice to support you in navigating your experience of gender and pregnancy.

Hold Your People Close

We know how important our community is, and it becomes extra vital while going through an experience as vulnerable as pregnancy. Now is the time to embrace your people—the ones who see you for who you truly are and will come support you if you are experiencing gender dysphoria or just really need someone to bring over a pint of ice cream.

Put Up Pictures of Other Queer/Trans Pregnant People

Representation matters. You are not the first genderqueer or trans pregnant person, and you definitely won't be the last. Even if you've never known any other pregnant people like you, you can find images on Instagram or other social media of pregnant queer and trans people. Print out those pictures and put them up in your home. Surrounding yourself with images of people like you going through similar experiences can do wonders in cutting the isolation that pregnant queer and trans people can sometimes experience.

Connect with Other Pregnant Trans or Genderqueer People

The internet is awesome for connecting with people we've never met before around shared experiences. There are Facebook groups, meetups led by queer doulas, and in-person gatherings where you can connect with other genderqueer and trans pregnant people. There are also some people who have been open on social media about their pregnancy experiences, and many of them are available to talk about what their experiences were like and hear about yours. Not feeling isolated is a very important part of your mental health. You'll find a list of trans pregnancy and lactation Facebook groups in the appendix on page 298.

Have a Therapist

While we realize that therapy, let alone therapy with an LGBTQ+-competent and affirming provider, is not accessible to everyone, we strongly recommend exploring your options. Having a safe place where you can process your feelings about your pregnancy is important. Find a therapist or counselor who can support you through all of it—the pregnancy stuff as well as the gender stuff.

Find an Affirming Provider

We've said it before and we'll say it again: Having a healthcare provider who understands and appreciates your experience of gender is hugely important as a genderqueer or trans pregnant person. You can interview your obstetrician or midwife about their experiences working with genderqueer and trans clients, and ask what training they've done to support genderqueer and trans people and whether or not they have an office environment that is safe and affirming.

For many genderqueer and/or trans people, the decision to become pregnant in the first place is complicated, and many fear that being pregnant will trigger challenging feelings of gender dysphoria. While this is the case for some, almost all of the previously pregnant genderqueer or trans folks we've spoken to about their experiences inevitably feel some element of pride in their bodies that grew and birthed their babies, queerly and in their own ways.

Following the evening I dashed through the rain with a cooler of dry ice and a tiny vial of washed sperm, I slept in the loft of a tiny, rented casita. There was barely enough room for me to sit up without bumping my head, but the skylight made the cramped space feel both cozy and expansive. I crossed my fingers and whisper wished to the moon that this one would stick. My hand rubbed clockwise circles around my belly, willing those sperm to swim and crack through one of my eggs.

I was superstitious about waiting until past the time I'd normally get my period before taking a pregnancy test. I'd been late before and none of the previous tries in ten cycles had stuck. So one afternoon when looking for secondhand furniture, I bought a pregnancy test and took it in a public bathroom. It sat on the window ledge, the boss of which direction my life would go next.

Pregnant!

It became the thing I was doing—like everything else was a detail laddering up to the moment I'd meet my child. I began a belly diary, which made me feel like I was channeling my inner tween girl. I noticed every gurgle, twinge, centimeter. That glow, it's a thing. My hair grew thick and long.

The first morning I woke up nauseous, I'd never been more excited to puke. I'd read about this being caused by pregnancy hormones, a sign that my little embryo was sticking. But the morning sickness lost its charm quickly. Within a matter of months, maybe weeks, I felt a shifting of hormones that not only brought on worse waves of morning sickness but impacted my experience of gender in a way that felt both liberating and ungrounding. Within my first trimester my belly grew noticeably on good food for that embryo that kept on sticking.

There were food cravings more demanding than when I was a teen. Ethiopian. Plain soft frozen yogurt with strawberry rhubarb topping. Kale salad with garlic croutons. More Ethiopian. Ben & Jerry's, you get the idea. My pants became too tight to button—I used hair ties to make an extended loop from my buttonhole to my button, wore flannel shirts and boots and carried that belly like a beer gut or a secret identity with a pocket full of almonds to abate the morning sickness. As my breasts grew, so did my cleavage and I played with how it felt to wear low-cut shirts in public— both vulnerable and womanly and strange.

Over time, my body felt better in pregnancy than before. There was a receding of both my sexuality and familiarity in my gender experience. I felt turned on and sometimes masturbated but had a hard time picturing how to bring in another person and stake space as a solo parent. I struggled to hold both my queerness and my pregnancy. I wondered how I was perceived. As my uterus stretched and my belly grew, I shopped both for men's pants and feminine tops and dresses.

I felt most myself when I was naked, without the presentation of clothes, laboring, surrounded by people who love me as I am, ready to welcome this new life into our apartment on Hawthorne Street in Brooklyn. —Katy Chatel

Expecting a Baby but Not Pregnant? This Section Is for You!

As a non-gestational parent with no biological relationship to my future baby, I feel a mixture of gratitude and grief. I've known since kindergarten—long before I came out as queer or trans—that I wanted to parent and did not want to be pregnant. I am lucky to be

partnered with someone who wanted to parent and be
pregnant. Witnessing their pregnancy has given me immense
appreciation for the physical sacrifices they are undergoing
to build our family. However, I also feel grief and fear that
our baby will more quickly and easily bond with my partner
than with me. I worry about being seen as less of a parent by
the various worlds we occupy and know that other people's
opinions could reinforce my own insecurities. I remain open
to being pleasantly surprised and proven wrong, but I'm also
fortifying my new-parent heart with connections to other
non-gestational parents with whom I can process any of the
tougher feelings that arise. —Asher

Those of you who are expecting a baby but aren't experiencing pregnancy have your own unique and valuable experiences that deserve to be honored. Whether you have a pregnant boo and are busy rubbing their feet, bringing them sparkling water, and comforting them when they start to cry during an insurance commercial, or are in communication with a surrogate on the other side of the country, you are still, in a nonphysical way, experiencing a type of gestation. Even though your future child isn't growing inside your body, your future child is growing, you are in the process of becoming a parent, and you deserve some loving attention for all that.

It can be easy for people's focus to go toward the pregnant person in the relationship or for friends and community members to not really know how to show up while you are expecting a baby through adoption or surrogacy. While some people appreciate that they don't need to do the work of gestating the child, others wish that they could do it, if only circumstances allowed. Some people may also feel grief about not being able to carry a pregnancy within their body due to the confines of their biology.

Wherever you land on this spectrum, we want to celebrate your impending parenthood and erase any doubt around your experience being just as legitimate as a pregnant person's. Also, you deserve support. We recommend reaching out to other folks you know who have had similar experiences and connecting with them as much as you can, or finding a support group for non-gestational parents. And make sure to honor yourself. Throw yourself some kind of queer baby shower that involves being seen and honored as the parent you are becoming. Or better yet, ask a friend to throw it for you.

We also recommend taking the time to think about your experience for when your baby is here, including postpartum support and feeding options. Plenty of non-gestational parents find ways to feed their babies that feel legitimizing and intimate, whether with their breasts, chest, or an SNS system. This can be an important way to bond with your child once they are here.

> A big part of my bonding with the twins was that I comfort-nursed them, and someone giving me permission to do that was huge for us. So I was like the human pacifier for them. Especially at the beginning when one was done eating but not sucking. Our lactation consultant at the hospital was like, "You can put the baby to your breast, too," and I was like, "I can?" and she said, "You have breasts, go for it." —Stephanie Hayes

Pregnancy (your own, your partner's, or your surrogate's) can be a roller coaster of intense emotions, new physical experiences, wild dreams, and deep spiritual significance. It can also be a time when all you can bear to do is sit on the couch watching *Queer Eye* and eat salt-and-vinegar chips.

We hope that this chapter provides you with some of the

information that you need to navigate through early pregnancy, whether it's happening inside your body or not. Again, we wish we could keep talking about everything throughout the entire pregnancy, including birth options, the postpartum period, lactation for everybody (who wants to), and so much more. But for now, please just take this: Whatever your experience of pregnancy is, it's normal, and you are not alone.

CHAPTER 8

Miscarriage and Infertility: When Things Don't Go as Planned

We took an at-home (pregnancy) test eleven days post-trigger-shot, five days post-transfer. It was faint, but there it was. A second line. We told "blasty" we loved her. We sent her warmth. We tried not to get excited; it was too early. The next day, we saw the line, just a little bit darker, but light bleeding had become a little heavier. We breathed. *It's okay.* I googled it—maybe this is implantation spotting?

Over the next two days cramps increased, blood darkened and got heavier. On the third day, there was still a line; it couldn't be a trigger shot, but I couldn't contemplate or understand the blood, trying to rationalize color and amounts, clots, and cramps. The line faded, lighter and lighter. We said goodbye to the blastocyst that had, if only for a moment, implanted inside of me. Chemical pregnancies can be harder when you are tracking your cycle, when you are with a clinic. Bleeding just a few days before or after your scheduled cycle would have begun; if you weren't looking, you would think it was your period.

We cried on the bathroom floor as I tried to remain hopeful and attempt to repress the grief that I so deeply needed to feel. Pregnancy test was negative, no sign of those two lines we had held on to for three days last week—I wonder if it was the trigger shot after all. Do we have permission to grieve this early loss? The next cycle started just a few days later. Back to monitoring, back to shots, back to blood tests and ultrasounds. —Laine Halpern Zisman

Most people don't pick up a book on family building and fertility imagining that miscarriage and infertility will be part of their own stories, but we'd be lying if we didn't acknowledge that things don't always go as planned. Some people get and stay pregnant relatively quickly, but others do not. Sometimes you, your partner, or your surrogate miscarries. Other times, months of inseminations and negative pregnancy tests pile up.

Ten to twenty percent of known pregnancies end in miscarriage, and it's estimated that one in eight people will experience fertility problems—a ratio that only seems to be increasing in modern times. Miscarriage and infertility are incredibly common experiences of childbearing people. It's a frequent grief, one that our culture is scared to talk about, which often leaves people experiencing infertility and miscarriage feeling very isolated.

For LGBTQ+ and solo people, this isolation can be even greater. We don't see ourselves represented in literature and discussions about infertility and loss, and the few resources available are geared toward families that don't look like ours. Additionally, the majority of pregnancies in our communities come with so much intentionality and hard work. The grief of an imagined future can be devastating. Hand in hand with that, of course, is the sense of scarcity when you lack easy access to gametes or financial resources, or you don't have the emotional support of a partner. Stress and concerns come with the constant decision-making and the time spent weighing pros and cons about future family building. Our community's burden in fertility struggles is often greater and unseen.

If you are going through these experiences, be it as a person trying to become pregnant yourself, a partner of someone who will carry the pregnancy, or someone growing their family through surrogacy, we hope this chapter offers you the information you need and some of the emotional support and resources that you deserve in navigating through the confusing, challenging waters of miscarriage and infertility. We are breaking this chapter into two sections—miscarriage, beginning next, and infertility, beginning on page 236.

MISCARRIAGE

In the broadest terms, miscarriage is the spontaneous loss of a pregnancy before twenty weeks. It can occur at any point during a pregnancy, but 80 percent of miscarriages occur in the first trimester. Miscarriage is incredibly common, perhaps surprisingly so given how little people talk about it: 10 to 20 percent of known pregnancies end in miscarriage, and the real rate of miscarriage may be as high as 50 percent, with most occurring so early that people didn't know they were pregnant.[1]

Knowing that miscarriage is a common experience doesn't make it any easier. Our culture is very scared of pregnancy loss—which adds to the isolation hopeful parents experience when moving through loss. Experiences of miscarriage and pregnancy loss can be incredibly heartbreaking and disappointing, and these feelings are often compounded by the close people in our lives' inabilities to support us through them.

We know that miscarriage as an LGBTQ+ and/or prospective solo parent can be even harder. As we detail throughout this book, both insemination using a sperm donor and the surrogacy process often come with a host of financial stressors and emotional and logistical challenges. There can be added stress and confusion regarding the question of changing your donor, conception method, or introducing medical interventions when things don't go as planned. Not to mention the fact that if we find any resources to support people through miscarriage, the vast majority of the time they are geared toward married, heterosexual individuals. Even without all the logistics LGBTQ+ and solo people have to contend with, the heartbreak of experiencing a miscarriage can be profound.

What Causes a Miscarriage?

The vast majority of miscarriages occur in the first trimester, and almost all are caused by genetic abnormalities in the growing fetus. Experiencing one or even two miscarriages doesn't necessarily mean that it will happen again. However, current guidelines recommend seeking fertility care after experiencing three or more consecutive miscarriages if you're under thirty-five, and two consecutive miscarriages if you're over thirty-five.

Miscarriages that occur in the second trimester can be caused by genetic issues, abdominal trauma, cervical insufficiency (when the cervix isn't strong enough to hold the pregnancy inside the uterus), infection, drug use, placental issues, and health issues in the parent or surrogate. Occasionally, miscarriages do have a root cause that can be treatable, such as autoimmune conditions or genetic mutations, and a care provider can help determine if there's a medical cause that can be treated to prevent further losses. No matter when someone experiences a pregnancy loss, regardless of the cause, it is not your fault. The reason that a person experiences miscarriage or pregnancy loss isn't a result of something they did or didn't do, and has no bearing on who they are as a person or what kind of parent they will become.

You Are Not Broken

Miscarriage is a normal experience for childbearing people, and the vast majority of miscarriages are entirely unpreventable. No, it wasn't because you drank three cups of coffee that day or you went for a run or you didn't tell your pregnant partner to stop working nights. We are not in control of every aspect of health and well-being, especially pregnancy. Even so, cultural silence around miscarriage often prompts people to worry that there's something wrong with them, and guilt for feeling jealous of the people around them who are having babies when they aren't.

Compounding the grief and heartbreak that comes with losing a pregnancy, miscarriage often has the potential to open the door for negative messages about people's bodies, vestiges of internalized homophobia, transphobia, sexism, and ableism. A lot of messages in society tell us that AFAB people's worth comes from their ability to carry a pregnancy, and ableism tells us if you miscarry or struggle to conceive, there's something wrong with you. For people who grew up in more homophobic environments, questions of if they deserve to become a parent, or if g-d is punishing them can emerge. There can be a deep feeling of being a failure because your body is not doing what it's "supposed" to be able to do. This is all BS, and if you are struggling with these feelings, we see you, and we encourage you to feel your grief but also, as much as possible, to try to leave society's problematic messaging behind.

What Happens During a Miscarriage?

When most people think of miscarriage, they imagine a spontaneous miscarriage: where a person notices spotting or bleeding in the hours or days prior, then progressive uterine cramping starts that pushes the body to miscarry the pregnancy. There are in fact a lot of different ways miscarriage can look, and in this section we will go through the five common scenarios that happen with miscarriage.

Chemical Pregnancy

A chemical pregnancy is a pregnancy that ends before five weeks. A person might have had a positive pregnancy test followed by a negative pregnancy test and/or an abnormally heavy period that comes a few days to a week later than expected. This may happen more often for folks like Laine (from page 210) who are utilizing IUI and IVF and take pregnancy tests very early, before the missed period. The passing of a chemical pregnancy is typically uncomplicated medically, but for people who have been trying to conceive a very desired pregnancy, it can be devastating.

The good news is that if you have experienced a chemical pregnancy while doing insemination methods such as ICI or IUI, you got the timing right—sperm and egg met and began forming a blastocyst. This means that chances are, if you continue inseminating around a similar time in future cycles, you are likely to conceive again, and hopefully this one will implant and continue to grow.

Spontaneous Miscarriage

A spontaneous miscarriage is where the body spontaneously and naturally expels a pregnancy that is no longer viable. A spontaneous miscarriage can start off feeling like getting a period, but cramps intensify. The emotions surrounding the cramping can also make the sensations harder to cope with. Once the body has passed the pregnancy, bleeding may remain heavy but should taper off significantly. It can be normal to experience some vaginal bleeding for a few weeks after the miscarriage, but bleeding should become progressively lighter with time.

Missed Miscarriage

Some people have a miscarriage diagnosed by ultrasound, when it is discovered that a fetus does not have a heartbeat. This is called a missed miscarriage. Most of these miscarriages happen between six to twelve weeks of pregnancy. A missed miscarriage can also occur in the second trimester, but this is extremely rare.

Threatened Miscarriage

Not all miscarriages are straightforward. Sometimes there is a period of threatened miscarriage when a baby is measuring small on ultrasound or a person is experiencing spotting or a questionable gush of fluid. This can be a time of heightened anxiety because of the uncertainty. Some threatened miscarriages become inevitable and the pregnancy passes, while others continue to grow into full-term healthy babies. Medically, the term *threatened miscarriage* refers to any vaginal bleeding before twenty weeks of pregnancy. About 50 percent of people who experience threatened miscarriage go on to birth healthy, full-term babies.[2]

Incomplete Miscarriage

Sometimes a pregnancy does not pass completely from the uterus, leaving the body trying to expel the remaining pieces with continued bleeding or spotting that does not resolve within a few weeks. This is an incomplete miscarriage, and if it's not caught and treated, it can lead to infection. An incomplete miscarriage often requires medical attention. We will detail the situations where it makes sense to get medical support in the following sections.

What Should I Know About Symptoms of Miscarriage?

All these different types of miscarriages can come with a range of physical experiences and stressors and require different kinds of interventions—ranging from monitoring at home to medical procedures to empty the uterus. Across the board, if a person miscarries it is normal for them to experience progressive cramping and heavy bleeding (soaking two large pads an hour for two hours), then pass the products of conception along with clots up to the size of a lemon, then see a quick shift to lighter bleeding after pregnancy passes.

We always recommend being in touch with your provider if you believe you are experiencing miscarriage symptoms to prevent complications from excessive blood loss. Seek immediate medical attention if...

You are soaking two large pads an hour for more than two hours, feeling light-headed or faint, or experiencing continued heavy bleeding for more than twenty-four hours.

You pass a clot larger than a lemon.

You feel a gush of fluid.

You experience miscarriage symptoms in the second trimester.

Medical Interventions for Miscarriage

In the event of a missed or incomplete miscarriage, the person miscarrying has the option to wait to pass the pregnancy naturally or use medical interventions to complete the miscarriage.

A miscarriage can be completed with a medication combo of mifepristone and misoprostol,[3] which will trigger the body to expel the pregnancy. This medication can be taken either as a suppository or orally and usually causes complete miscarriage within twenty-four hours. It's safe, it's noninvasive, and it allows people to remain home to pass a pregnancy. It does, however, cause painful cramping that can last up to twenty-four hours.

A miscarriage can also be completed with a procedure like dilation and curettage (D&C) or dilation and extraction (D&E). During a D&C, a doctor uses a sterile tool to dilate the cervix and scrape the uterine walls to remove the contents of the uterus; in a D&E, the doctor dilates the cervix and then aspirates the uterine contents. Both procedures are usually performed under some type of sedation and/or numbing medication. The benefit of a D&C or a D&E is that both are relatively quick procedures. It usually only takes about five to fifteen minutes, depending on how far along the pregnancy was. The drawbacks (for some people) are that it can feel very clinical and can also be uncomfortable, depending on the sedation options provided by the doctor.

It is also possible to wait for a missed miscarriage to pass spontaneously—as long as there is no significant bleeding, signs of infection, or any other causes for concern. Waiting for a missed miscarriage to pass spontaneously is called expectant management, and it usually completes within two to six weeks. Eighty percent of people doing expectant management will complete a normal miscarriage at home.[4] Some folks take herbs such as parsley or cotton root bark extract to encourage the uterus to release its contents. If expectant management doesn't yield a complete miscarriage, doctors recommend taking medication or having a D&C to avoid infection or a rare condition called disseminated intravascular coagulation.

Second-Trimester Miscarriages

Miscarriages after the first trimester are much less common, with only about 2 to 4 percent occurring in the second trimester. Miscarriage after twelve weeks of pregnancy may also be called a fetal demise and can be discovered by absence of fetal heart tones in a prenatal appointment or by symptoms like bleeding, cramping, or a gush of fluid. Depending on the gestational age, people's options may include mifepristone and misoprostol, a D&C or D&E procedure, or a process similar to a labor induction.

TERMINATING WANTED PREGNANCIES

Sometimes people terminate wanted pregnancies, due to either anomalies discovered in the fetus from genetic screening that are incompatible with life, or health issues in the pregnant person that are too great to manage while pregnant or become life-threatening. There is a unique and isolating grief in having to make a decision to end a desired pregnancy. And in a post-Roe America, this can create sometimes impossible hurdles to accessing medically necessary care to prevent pain, suffering, and death in the parent.

Follow-Up Medical Care

Follow-up care after a miscarriage is essential in order to confirm that the pregnancy has completely passed. This can be done by blood test or ultrasound with a midwife or a doctor. Folks with a negative blood type need to be given a RhoGAM injection within seventy-two hours of the start of bleeding to prevent complications with future pregnancies due to the risk of Rh sensitization.

WHAT IS RH SENSITIZATION?

People with a negative blood type lack a certain protein in their blood cells that is present in the cells of people with a positive blood type. If someone with a negative blood type (Rh-negative) gets pregnant with a fetus with a positive blood type (Rh-positive), there is a slight chance that their blood could mix during a miscarriage (or during labor). If this happens, the Rh-negative person's blood may recognize the unfamiliar protein of the Rh-positive blood as an invader, which can cause their body to attack future pregnancies, resulting in recurrent miscarriages.

For pregnant people with Rh-negative blood, it's standard to receive a shot called RhoGAM, which effectively immunizes them against reacting to Rh-positive blood. The recommendation is to receive a shot of RhoGAM in the event of a miscarriage as well as at twenty-eight weeks of pregnancy and within seventy-two hours of giving birth to an Rh-positive baby.[5]

Trying Again

From a medical perspective, there is no "right" time to start trying to conceive again after experiencing miscarriage. Some people will feel ready to start trying again right away—others will need a few months (or more) to grieve their loss before trying to conceive again.

Some people find it helpful to talk with a midwife or doctor after a miscarriage to check in about their health and receive support or guidance. Recurrent miscarriage—experiencing three or more miscarriages under age thirty-five or two or more miscarriages over thirty-five—can be a sign of health issues that impact fertility. This can be a good time to seek care from a gynecologist or fertility specialist to investigate possible causes. For people with uteruses, that can include ultrasounds for fibroids and uterine anomalies; labs for thyroid function, diabetes, hormones, autoimmune conditions, and thrombophilic conditions that affect the ability to stay pregnant; genetic screening; and evaluation for pelvic inflammatory disease. For people with sperm, this can include semen analysis and genetic screening.

I knew that there is a surge in fertility after miscarriage, but when my LH surged eleven days after my miscarriage, I was not prepared. The sperm bank I was using was in my city, so I called and paid an extra $40 fee to get my sperm out the next morning, then hustled across town between work meetings for my midwife to fit me in for an IUI in between appointments. It was so stressful, and I felt desperate. When I got my period two weeks later, I kinda lost it. I realized I needed to take a break for a month or two to just be sad. —Rachel

Sometimes moving through miscarriage makes folks want to change conception plans. Our general rule of thumb is if you've tried something three to six times and it hasn't worked, switch up some part of the plan. That may mean switching up donors, inseminating earlier or later in the cycle, or changing insemination methods. If you're considering switching something up, we recommend returning to the decision tree on page 16 and reconsidering your plan from where you are now.

Remember, if you need to, you can always decide to take a short break from trying to conceive to reevaluate your choices and process your feelings. Some people may want to take a break from trying, and others will want to double down and try and get pregnant again immediately. If you're needing something to be different after a loss, listen to that need.

A NOTE ON FOLIC ACID

Many people know about taking folic acid to prevent fetal abnormalities that can cause miscarriage, but did you know that some people can't actually metabolize folic acid? Folic acid is the synthetic version of folate, aka vitamin B_9, which converts to 5-MTHF in the digestive system. Since folic acid is made in a lab, it takes more work for the body to metabolize folic acid in the liver, whereas folate, the natural form, is more easily absorbed in the digestive tract.[6]

You can take a genetic test that determines whether or not you have a gene called MTHFR, which is a common gene mutation. If you do have this gene (like Marea does), the process of metabolizing folic acid in the liver is even less effective.[7] A folate or methylated B-vitamin supplement can remedy this issue.

Whether or not you get tested for MTHR, if you're planning to try to carry a pregnancy again, we recommend taking a prenatal vitamin with at least 400mcg of folate. You can also find folate in foods like dark leafy vegetables, beans, nuts, whole grains, liver, and eggs.

Coping with Grief and Loss

The emotional experiences following miscarriage are as diverse as the people experiencing them. Some people feel profound sadness; others do not. Some people grieve the pregnancy loss as a child; others grieve a more ambiguous loss of possibility and an imagined future. When Ray lost their pregnancy, they were completely caught off guard by how intense the aftermath was. It went beyond feeling sad—something they had wanted so badly and worked so hard toward had come to fruition and then had gone away so quickly.

For people who have experienced a miscarriage before they told many people that they were pregnant, it can be especially challenging to give themselves permission to grieve and to seek support. Sharing the news and the heartbreak in one fell swoop can be a lot to ask of yourself.

No matter what you find yourself feeling, embrace it. And if you need permission to grieve, consider it granted. Take the time and space you need. Even the simplest actions, like allowing yourself to cry when you feel sad, are quite literally healing. Yes, really! Crying triggers the body to produce oxytocin and endorphins,[8] which helps release emotional pain. It's healthy to grieve, and crying helps process a grief experience on a cellular level. For folks who have a hard time accessing grief, getting professional care can help. It's also supportive for some people to get the tears flowing by watching something you know helps you cry (like *The Lion King* for Marea, and people in the military coming home to pets videos for Ray).

Journaling, or seeking professional support through individual therapy, can provide a safe, nonjudgmental space to process your thoughts and emotions after loss, and therapists can also support you in deciding on next steps around conception or family creation and help you process any feelings that may come up during future pregnancies. We talk more about stress-reduction tools that may be useful to you during this time on page 86 as well as on page 125.

We also frequently recommend that our clients seek out support groups to counteract the feeling of isolation that is so common with miscarriage. There are groups on Facebook available for LGBTQ+ and solo parents trying to conceive and some that specifically address pregnancy loss. Organizations like Our Family Coalition and Single Mothers by Choice may also offer support groups that may address your needs. You can find more resources at the back of this book and on our website, www.babymakingforeverybody.com.

Experiencing Miscarriage as a Non-Gestational Parent

Non-gestational parents, partners, and people using surrogates also experience a range of emotions with miscarriage, holding not only their own grief about loss of the pregnancy but also a deep compassion for their partner's or their surrogate's physical pain.

The sense of powerlessness around their family formation hopes, and in not being able to take the previously pregnant person's pain away or support them more during the process, can be equally crushing, though as a society we tend to focus our attention on the individual who miscarried, rather than thinking about the family system involved. As a result, non-gestational parents may also feel invisible in a miscarriage process, with the physical needs and experiences of the person who carried the pregnancy overtaking their own feelings of grief.

If the gestational parent or surrogate needs to access medical care for the miscarriage, partners or biological parents may experience invisibility heightened by homophobic and transphobic assumptions about relationships in mainstream healthcare settings. If you find yourself in this situation, it can be helpful to have a doula or a friend there with you to help hold space for you and advocate on your behalf to the medical staff, or process after the fact.

Miscarriage grief can also lead to challenges in relationships as each person moves through their own process differently. This has the potential to cause extra sadness for the partner of someone going through a miscarriage and bring some fear or internalized homophobia and/or transphobia about not being the "real" parent, which, we just want to say, is completely untrue.

It can be challenging to find the balance between supporting your partner and getting your own support, but we want to say loud and clear that your experience matters! Even if you weren't carrying the pregnancy, even if you weren't biologically related to this child who is no longer, your experience matters. It is wonderful and loving that you want to support your partner or your surrogate, especially if the hard thing is happening in their body. AND. We want to offer a friendly reminder that you deserve support as well.

Supporting Yourself as the Non-Gestational Parent

If your partner is experiencing a miscarriage, the person you typically lean on for support might not be as available to support you. It can be a tough balancing act, and we want to say again that your needs and experience matter, and you don't have to be alone with this. Miscarriage is an incredibly common experience, and if you know anyone whose partner or surrogate has gone through a miscarriage and you feel comfortable doing so, give them a call. Or find a support group for LGBTQ+ pregnancy loss. If you can contact the organizer of such a group and let them know that you're looking to talk to other people in a similar situation, there's a good chance that they will connect you with other folks who are also interested in talking about this topic.

We know we've said this a million times throughout this book, but we want to reiterate that therapy can be immensely helpful. People process grief and loss in their own ways, and it is important to get individual support to help move through loss in the healthiest way possible. If you do not have access to therapy, journaling or support groups can also be wonderful resources. If you find that you want or need support in a relational context, we strongly recommend looking to a family therapist. You can screen for providers who are LGBTQ+-friendly, and many therapists are able to work on a sliding scale.

You and your partner or surrogate may have differences in conception plans or desires following miscarriage. Have open-ended conversations about family-planning wishes. Try to notice your desires before coming into a conversation, because grief sometimes leads to black-and-white thinking, which can look like more reactive conversations and less skills in listening and flexibility.

When working with a surrogate, we encourage families to have conversations before conception about how everyone would like to handle a potential pregnancy loss. It's impossible to know how you, your partner, or a surrogate would feel in the moment, so be open to plans changing. But it is really helpful to begin these conversations before beginning the trying to conceive process.

Our surrogate for our first baby experienced a stillbirth at twenty weeks, which was due to an extremely rare cord accident. The experience was profoundly traumatic all around. After the loss, our doctors recommended that we use a different surrogate, but we felt loyal to her. So after six months of waiting for her body to heal, we did another transfer, and the embryo stuck.

After the loss, I was extremely anxious when she got pregnant again. My husband, on the other hand, felt like it was going to work out this time: that it was meant to be. But both our surrogate and I were pretty anxious the entire time. I tried a lot of coping mechanisms: Meditation helped, as did therapy, but I did still have a sense of anxiety. Luckily, nine months later, we ended up with a beautiful, amazing son. Looking back, it does feel meant to be—this is the child we were meant to raise. —Neill Sullivan

INFERTILITY

While miscarriage marks the loss of a potential future, infertility can feel like endless limbo. All the lifestyle changes, the tracking, the conception attempts, doctors, decision-making, and piles of negative pregnancy tests are overwhelming to say the least. It can feel like holding your breath waiting for the next chapter of your life to start, and then month after month never coming up for air. Experiencing infertility can look like having multiple miscarriages in a row or trying to get pregnant month after month without getting a positive pregnancy test.

> I am part of a club that I never signed up for or wanted to join, but the dues I am paying for this group come in the form of hundreds and thousands of dollars, heartache, heartbreak, knowing that my body is failing me and that there is nothing I can do about it. I am infertile, but that's not my only problem—I am an infertile lesbian who has a healthcare plan that doesn't account for me. —Lola & Mush

Just like miscarriage, infertility is incredibly common in our society—one in eight people who are trying to conceive experience fertility problems. One of the challenges of navigating infertility as LGBTQ+ people and prospective solo parents is that the standards are designed around cisgender, heterosexual couples. In other words, infertility and infertility treatments are defined and researched with the assumption that the individuals involved have a uterus, eggs, and abundant access to sperm in their relationship and can make regular, reasonably well-timed attempts at conception. Within this construct, infertility is defined as trying to conceive without a viable pregnancy for six months for people with uteruses over thirty-five, and for a year for people with uteruses under thirty-five. The age of the person with sperm isn't accounted for.

While some queer and solo parents do certainly experience infertility, it's not clear from this definition that the diagnosis applies to our bodies. What if we're accessing "infertility" treatments as conception tools from the first try? What if every insemination was well timed? Or if some conception experiences occurred at home and others within a fertility clinic? What if we're only using frozen sperm? These are ways that the "infertility" diagnosis parameters don't fit many LGBTQ+ or solo prospective parents' experiences, and as a result, the infertility care and interventions do not quite fit our needs or experiences.

As we move through the following section, we'll be talking about the different reasons people can have a hard time creating a pregnancy and the interventions available to treat these different scenarios. As we mentioned above, the trigger for evaluation and intervention is based on cisgender, heterosexual couples' needs and experiences. Since we don't yet have an LGBTQ+- or solo-parent-centered standard for understanding fertility and infertility, we are going to utilize (with a critical eye) the definitions, tools, and data we have available right now from mainstream infertility care. The standards of care aren't designed for us, so we need to sit with our needs and the experiences of our bodies and make the decisions that work for us.

What Is Infertility?

Because we don't yet have an LGBTQ+- or solo-parent-centered definition, we are going to consider the diagnosis for infertility as trying to conceive without a pregnancy for twelve months if the uterus-haver is under thirty-five, and for six months when over thirty-five. However, as midwives serving the LGBTQ+ and solo parent community, we also hold this definition loosely. We consider fertility to be the presence of normal fertility signs that indicate the ability to conceive and creating a pregnancy within a reasonable time frame for your mind, body, and spirit. With this caveat in mind, some of our clients will access infertility care after four months of trying—others will wait two years to access more in-depth medical care.

When a person meets the traditional diagnostic criteria for infertility, it doesn't mean they cannot get pregnant; however, it does mean their chances of conception are lower—statistically about a 5 percent chance of conceiving per cycle without adding infertility interventions.[9] Recurrent miscarriages—experiencing two or more miscarriages in a row—is considered subfertility, not infertility.

However, many of the same infertility evaluations and treatments are used in cases of people experiencing recurrent miscarriages.

As we know, there are three ingredients required in creating a pregnancy—sperm, eggs, and a uterus. So, if there's something amiss in any of these three ingredients, it's possible to experience infertility. Larger health issues, like diabetes, clotting disorders, and cancer, can also interfere with fertility because fertility is connected to all of our body's systems/organs. In the following sections, we will go over the considerations for all types of infertility and how to access care for each.

If You're a Person with Sperm...

Infertility for people assigned male at birth comes down, essentially, to two things—issues with the number of sperm in an ejaculate or difficulties in the body's ability to transport sperm from the testicles. In cisgender heterosexual couples, about 40 to 50 percent of infertility is caused by sperm issues.[10]

There are two terms used to identify people experiencing diminished sperm production. The most common is *oligospermia*, which literally means low sperm count—this impacts about 2 percent of all people with sperm[11] and 40 percent of people with sperm who are experiencing infertility or suboptimal fertility.[12] People with oligospermia have less than fifteen million sperm per milliliter of semen (by comparison, average sperm count is fifteen million to two hundred million per milliliter). Its more extreme cousin, *azoospermia*, which is when a person is not producing sperm, affects roughly 10 to 15 percent of AMAB people experiencing infertility.[13]

Both oligospermia and azoospermia can be caused by chromosomal defects, hormonal differences, past infection or injury, immune disorders, some medications (such as steroids, some cancer medications, and certain antibiotics[14]), or structural issues like a varicocele (an enlargement of the veins in the scrotum). Varicoceles are present in about 40 percent of fertility problems involving people with sperm and can be corrected by surgery.

Differences in hormone levels can also affect sperm count. Some of these differences may be part of a person's unique hormone picture, including lower testosterone, insensitivity to androgens, and high prolactin level; and others can be caused by gender-affirming hormone therapy. You can find more information about low sperm counts for AMAB people in chapter 5. Environmental factors play a huge role in sperm production and quality, with exposure to alcohol, drugs, tobacco, environmental toxins, or excessive heat negatively affecting sperm quality.

The other cause of infertility in people with sperm is issues with transporting sperm from the testicles. About 10 to 20 percent of sperm factor infertility is caused by transport issues.[15] This can be caused by blockages in the transport tubes, which can be the result of past injury, scar tissue from surgery or past STI inflammation, or genetic differences. The shape of sperm (aka morphology), and the way they move (aka motility), can also make it difficult for sperm to travel and cause transport-related infertility.

You may have one of the risk factors listed above for low sperm count or a sperm transport issue but experience no signs or symptoms. If you have been trying to conceive with your sperm and it hasn't been working, or you would like more information about your fertility or a donor's fertility as part of decision-making, a semen analysis is the next step. You can schedule an appointment for a semen analysis with a primary care provider, with a fertility doctor, or through a sperm bank.

If you discover that your sperm count is under fifteen million, the next step is a more extensive workup with a fertility doctor. Evaluation for the causes of low or abnormal sperm includes reviewing medical and social history, lab work for hormone levels and different conditions that can impact sperm, and a physical exam for structural issues.

Treatments for low sperm counts can include medication like Clomid or human chorionic gonadotropin, surgery to correct a varicocele, or treating infections and other preexisting health conditions. For conception assistance, people with low sperm counts or abnormal morphology may use insemination tools like IUI and IVF, or utilize IVF with ICSI or extracting sperm via biopsy for conception with a very low sperm count. The larger list of current infertility interventions can be found on page 236.

If You're a Person with a Uterus...

Understanding infertility in people with eggs can be a bit more complex—socially, diagnostically, emotionally, and physically. AFAB people in reproductive health settings have a long history of not being listened to, and some folks may feel fear or anxiety come up when they need to access infertility care. There are also some messages from society that equate the worth of AFAB people with their ability to reproduce. Even if people don't agree with these oppressive ideas, they can still get into our subconscious and affect us psychologically when dealing with infertility. At the same time, infertility care has become quite a moneymaking industry in the US—some of the tools utilized in clinic settings are invasive, and many are very expensive.

There are causes of infertility that affect ovulation and available eggs, and others that affect the uterus. We'll be talking about the two concurrently in this section.

Unexplained infertility is surprisingly—and kind of infuriatingly—the most common form of infertility for AFAB individuals. About one in four[16] cases of infertility are unexplained, meaning that a fertility doctor can find no medical reason to explain why pregnancy isn't occurring.

The truth is that I had believed that if I was healthy, I would just get pregnant. I believed that because I don't have any major health issues, because I was a farmer for seven years and only ate organic food, because my hormones are well balanced, my fallopian tubes are clear, because I have regular periods, because I exercise, because, because, because, I should get pregnant. I had to face these thoughts for what they truly were—ableism.

Ableism is both a product of, and perpetuated by, capitalism and the hierarchical productivity-based society we live in in the US. One of the most insidious elements of ableist thinking is the idea that if you "take care of your health" you are in a way owed certain things, by your own body or by society. —Ellie Lobovits

Hormonal Causes

Let's start with a quick refresher about hormones. Normal hormone cycling happens over the course of a twenty-one- to thirty-six-day cycle starting with menstruation. The low levels of hormones during bleeding trigger the brain to produce FSH, which triggers the ovary to produce estrogen to get an egg ready to be released. When estrogen and FSH reach the right concentration in the bloodstream, it triggers the brain to produce LH. All of these hormones keep rising until they reach the perfect concentration, and then LH shoots up and causes an egg to release twenty-four to thirty-six hours later. FSH, LH, and estrogen drop off and progesterone, which is being produced by the ovary, rises to get the uterus ready. Progesterone triggers the ovary to help out with estrogen, and the two continue to rise for ten to twelve days until they realize there's no fertilized egg helping with hormones, and then drop off suddenly, triggering menstruation.

Hormone-based infertility issues interfere with this feedback cycle, preventing ovulation from happening or causing ovulation to occur infrequently in a way that makes it difficult to track fertility and time inseminations. This causes more difficulty in conceiving. Hormone-based infertility can be diagnosed through home cycle tracking or lab work. Signs of anovulatory cycles, aka lack of ovulation, include cycles under twenty days or longer than thirty-seven, frequent spotting, light or pale period bleeding, no temperature shifts or multiple temperature shifts over a long cycle, and high LH readings for many days.

Anovulatory cycles can be caused by PCOS, thyroid disorders, very low or high body weight, and exposure to endocrine disruptors, menopause, and other forms of high metabolic stress. We'll go into more detail on a few of the primary causes.

PCOS

Polycystic ovarian syndrome is one of the most common causes of infertility in people assigned female at birth.[17] It's a condition in which the ovaries produce an abnormal amount of androgens, which are sex hormones typically found in bodies assigned male at birth. PCOS is a biological variation of gender, which is possibly one of the reasons why it is seen at higher rates in the LGBTQ community. Some people notice symptoms of PCOS—facial hair, weight distribution, elevated blood sugar, and irregular cycles—and some do not. The elevated levels of testosterone and metabolic stress of high blood sugar prevent normal hormone cycling and impede ovulation, therefore decreasing a person's chance of conceiving each cycle.

Thyroid Issues

Hyperthyroidism, when the body produces too much thyroid hormone, and hypothyroidism, when the body produces too little thyroid hormone, are linked with infertility. The thyroid plays a key role in hormone production in the body, so when thyroid hormones are off, there's a good chance other hormones will be off as well. Signs of these conditions include longer-than-normal or shorter-than-normal periods, rapid weight loss or weight gain, and abnormally high or low energy, brittle hair/nails, and muscle tremors, among other things.[18] Both conditions are easily diagnosed with a blood test, which can be ordered by a primary care physician, midwife, ob-gyn, fertility specialist, or endocrinologist and treated with medication.

Ovarian Issues

Sometimes ovaries stop producing enough estrogen, the hormone necessary for ovulation. It's common for these hormones to decrease as we age, but when this happens before the age of forty, it's called premature ovarian insufficiency. This affects about one in one hundred people AFAB ages thirty through thirty-nine.

Structural Causes

If ovulation is occurring normally, it may be that a structural challenge is impacting the ability for egg and sperm to meet or for a fertilized egg to reach or implant in the uterus. Following are the most common causes.

Scarring in the Uterus or Fallopian Tubes

People who have a history of pelvic surgery, untreated pelvic inflammatory disorder, or a history of some sexually transmitted infections sometimes experience residual scarring in their uterus or fallopian tubes, which can block the egg's ability to travel into the uterus or prevent implantation.

Fibroids

A fibroid is a non-cancerous tumor that grows in the uterus. Large or plentiful uterine fibroids can sometimes impede implantation and are linked to infertility, either blocking a fertilized egg from reaching the uterus or leaving less room to implant. Fibroids don't always cause fertility issues. They are extremely common, with estimates that up to 68.6 percent[19] of AFAB people have fibroids (for reference, about 10 percent of AFAB people experience infertility).

Many people who have fibroids do not experience any symptoms, but some do. Symptoms include heavy periods, periods lasting longer than seven days, pelvic pain and pressure, bladder and constipation issues, and back and leg pain. The presence of fibroids is diagnosed via ultrasound, and if someone has multiple large fibroids, their doctor may recommend surgical removal prior to trying to conceive. Removing fibroids can increase pregnancy rates significantly.[20]

Bifurcated Uterus or Other Creative Uterine Shapes

Although this isn't a main cause of infertility, some people have a bifurcated uterus or other conditions known as uterine anomalies that can cause issues getting pregnant or maintaining a pregnancy. Researchers think that about 5 percent of all AFAB people have creatively shaped uteruses and have found these conditions in about 25 percent of people with a history of miscarriages or preterm deliveries.[21]

Endometriosis

Endometriosis is a condition in which small amounts of uterine tissue grow outside the uterus, such as in the fallopian tubes, causing pain and sometimes infertility. Symptoms of endometriosis include pain in the pelvis, back, bladder, and rectum that worsens during menstruation, pain with sex, long heavy periods, and gastrointestinal problems. Endometriosis affects about 10 percent[22] of AFAB people of reproductive age.

A NOTE ABOUT STRESS

It's extremely common for people struggling to conceive to hear that they need to "de-stress." This advice is about as helpful as you might think, and contrary to popular opinion, the research on stress and infertility has mixed results.[23] It seems unlikely that stress alone can cause infertility, and it is a challenging feeling to control for in the research. There is some research showing that people with a history of depression struggle with infertility at higher rates.[24] While we do know that stress and mental health are connected to fertility, we still don't know exactly how. Even so, a lot of fertility and infertility counseling is centered on stress reduction techniques, which can cause people to believe their fertility challenges are their fault.

That said, infertility itself is stressful, and stress-reduction techniques are beneficial in helping you support mental health, enjoy life outside of trying to conceive, and make decisions from a more centered place. Stress reduction can also support minimizing the coping tools folks use when stressed—not sleeping at night, eating for blood sugar spikes, lots of caffeine—that do affect fertility.

The biggest reminder we can offer is that infertility is stressful and not your fault. We do love for folks to have stress-reduction tools available to them when going through the highs and lows of infertility. Find and use the tools that bring you ease and not more anxiety.

What Do You Do if You're Experiencing Infertility?

There's no one right answer for how to make decisions when you're navigating infertility or potential infertility. We are not fertility doctors, and when we talk to clients who meet the diagnostic criteria for infertility, we recommend they consult with reproductive endocrinologists (aka fertility docs) to get more information about their health and utilize bigger tools.

If you have access to fertility care, it is important that you take the time to find a provider with whom you feel safe and can have compassionate conversations about options. We discuss tools for finding an LGBTQ+- or solo-parent-affirming provider on page 127. Once you're under care, it's typical to start with a fertility workup (described in chapter 4) and then review options and statistical chances of conception with each option available.

Options you might discuss with your provider are included below. We denote treatments focused on sperm with a (✦), treatments focused on eggs with a (✱), and treatments focused on uteruses with a (➔).

- Treating medical conditions contributing to infertility (say, with thyroid medication). (✦ ✱ ➔)
- Medication to treat hormone disorders for sperm quality. (✦)
- Ovulation monitoring and trigger shots to shorter ovulation window for home insemination, ICI or IUI. (✱)
- Surgery to treat varicocele to improve sperm production or to retrieve sperm. (✦)
- Intracytoplasmic sperm injection (ICSI) with IVF to inject a single sperm into an egg. (✦ ✱)
- Medication to stimulate ovulation for home or clinic insemination. (✱ ✦)
- Surgery to remove fibroids, uterine septum, or endometriosis. (✱)
- IVF with different medication regimens. (✦ ✱)
- IVF using different sperm or eggs. (✦ ✱)
- Genetic testing of embryos and embryo selection. (✦ ✱)

We want to acknowledge that cost is often a prohibitive factor in accessing infertility care in a medical setting or fertility clinic. Many insurance plans don't cover infertility care, and many in our community don't have insurance in the first place. Even for folks whose insurance plans do cover fertility services, LGBTQ+ and solo parents may not technically meet their criteria for accessing services since, again, the definitions were not made for us. The structure of capitalism and a for-profit medical industry limits people's reproductive choices by making accessing infertility care a privilege and limiting options for forming families.

For people who don't have insurance coverage for fertility clinics, a good deal of infertility testing can be ordered by a primary care provider, urologist, midwife, or ob-gyn. When you make an appointment, be clear with your provider about what you are looking for and your situation with your insurance, and be prepared to discuss the following:

For people with testes[25]

- Semen analysis.
- Blood work: testosterone, FSH, LH, prolactin STI testing, genetic testing, and karyotyping if low sperm count present.
- Post-ejaculation urinalysis.
- Physical exam, reviewing medications with provider, and ultrasound of scrotum, rectum, and testes.

For people with uteruses

- Blood work: complete blood count, hemoglobin A1C. Thyroid labs: TPO, reverse T3, TSH, free T4, blood type and Rh antibodies, folate, STI. Anticoagulant and lupus labs for people with recurrent miscarriages.
- Cycle day 3 hormone labs: estradiol, FSH, LH.
- Cycle day 21 (or seven days after ovulation): progesterone.

- Ultrasound: fibroids, endometriosis, polyps, follicles, uterine shape anomalies.
- Some OB offices can do an in-office saline sonogram to check fallopian tubes.

Some fertility surgeries like varicocele, fibroid removal, or endometriosis laparoscopy can be covered by general health insurance when they are performed for reasons other than infertility. In addition to treating health conditions that can affect fertility like thyroid disorders or elevated blood sugar, primary care providers can prescribe medications like letrozole or Clomid to induce ovulation or increase sperm count. While there are benefits to using these medications with monitoring from a fertility clinic, they are affordable on their own and can be accessed through primary care.

In cases where care is not accessible, many people consider creating their family in other ways, such as continuing with home inseminations, seeking pieces of infertility treatment from their primary care doctor or from low-cost health clinics, changing uteruses (when available) or sperm sources, or switching plans to fostering and adoption.

I have an initial consultation scheduled with a low-cost IVF clinic next month. And I'm excited for it, a sentiment I never thought I would feel. IVF used to seem like the big bad wolf at the end of a dark, dark road. It was for people who had fertility issues, who had hormonal issues, who were older than me, who had waited too long. In other words, not me.

Yes, IVF can be prohibitively expensive. IVF is somewhat invasive and relies on lots of hormones. Yes, many reproductive clinics are part of what I think of as the "fertility-industrial complex." Yes, considering IVF can feel like you are an alien on a strange planet where suddenly your body doesn't work and you need machines and drugs to take over. All of these things are true. And all of these things can bring up valid feelings of upset, sadness, and anger. I know they have for me.

And yet.

After five IUIs, over a dozen ultrasounds, multiple blood tests, taking hormones almost every day for two cycles, and the absolute roller coaster of emotions each month without one pregnancy, I realized I wanted to try a method that at least doubled if not tripled my chances of conceiving. I was done with the feelings of ableist shame that had arisen for me earlier, almost, it seems, a lifetime ago, when I had first considered IVF. —Ellie Lobovits

Separate from any conversation with a provider, we encourage you to take the time to sit with yourself and write out what feels most important in the sea of infertility options. There are no right or wrong paths, no matter what you choose. The most important thing is to center your priorities in pursuing parenthood. Speak with those in your close support system, and your partner(s) if applicable, and consider asking questions like:

- How important is it to you to have a child who is genetically related to you?
- What is your budget?
- What is your timeline to build your family?
- What level of medicalization are you up for?

Go back to your reflections about your priorities in forming a family from chapter 1. As you sit with your priorities and your experience in trying to conceive, what comes up? What options would allow you to center your priorities and values? What, if anything, do you want to revise?

It can be easy to get swept up in the gravity of the infertility care industry, but our hope for you is that you feel empowered to make your own decisions, even if these aren't decisions you hoped to have to make.

Embracing All the Feels

There comes a point in some journeys through infertility when we need to grapple with the unwanted reality. Sometimes, no matter how hard we try or how much we want it, things don't work out. This can be especially heartbreaking when it comes to our dreams of being pregnant and/or creating a family in a certain way, and it may feel impossible to let go of something that we have wanted so intensely for so long.

When we asked community members what advice they wished they had received when experiencing their own infertility journeys, we heard this again and again: Sometimes people don't need you to be hopeful for them. Sometimes they need you to sit with them and just accept the sh*ttiness of the situation.

Similar to those grieving miscarriage, people experiencing infertility often feel lost and isolated. Going through hard things alone can make it even harder. Finding a support group, whether it's online or just meeting with a friend or acquaintance whom you know has had a similar experience, can be an essential step in feeling less alone.

If you're uncomfortable speaking with a friend or don't have anyone in your network, consider speaking with a therapist. You can find a therapist in your area who specializes in pregnancy loss or infertility, as well as people who work closely with the LGBTQ+ and/or solo parent community. Make sure to take the time to find someone you feel comfortable with and with whom you feel deeply accepted.

Journaling can also be a wonderful support: Creating a safe space for yourself will help you process all your emotions, even the ones you don't feel comfortable saying out loud. More ideas for self-care in this process can be found on page 125.

When you're going through something as hard as infertility, it can be all-consuming and easy to lose touch with other aspects of life that bring happiness and connection. We encourage folks to find joy in life, even in small things like cuddling with a pet or going for a walk with a friend. Pursue goals outside of becoming a parent, and don't forget to take care of yourself, even when you feel like life just sucks. A day trip to the nearest body of water, going to a concert, or simple pleasures like indulging in a favorite comfort food can make a difference.

> Before our first IUI, I told my partner, "I think this one's going to work!" I had intuition that conception would be super fast and easy. One and a half years later, my tune had changed. I stopped believing that it was possible for us to ever see a second line on the pregnancy test. I started dreading the tests, because I knew that each one would pile on a new disappointment. —Asher

Infertility Is Not Your Fault

It's common for people struggling with infertility to feel that they have failed in some profound way. But you have not failed. There is nothing wrong with you. You are a good person with a good body. Many people who struggle with infertility cannot pinpoint why they aren't able to conceive. Whatever your situation, please try not to blame yourself and internalize infertility as some sort of personal failure.

In the beginning, my wife and I did as many things as we could think of to prepare to welcome a child into our family. During the preparation phase before our first insemination attempt, the labor of queer family making felt powerful and intentional. I felt hopeful and a closeness with my own body.

As we moved through several rounds of unsuccessful attempts, the hopefulness turned into heaviness and sadness. First came the intake forms that completely erased our identities (and those of single people trying to conceive). The titles *mother* and *father* were listed on all the forms to register us with our clinic (this clinic is one of the very few options in our geographic region). I crossed out all the *father*s. No one said anything when I turned in the forms, no apology, no acknowledgment. Then, as negative pregnancy tests accumulated, new questions arose: How long do we go with this method? (IUI is what we started with.) How much can we afford? When or do we switch to other methods? When do we move toward adoption? How do we care for our waiting? How do we tend to our sadness with compassion? I felt kind of suspended in time. We decided to pause for a few months to catch up with ourselves.

As I write this, there is still much to do, paths to choose, and the unknown to wade through. I am writing this from the murky middle. I don't know yet what my/our limits are of medical intervention, resources, and energy. I don't know if parenthood via pregnancy will happen, or if we will initiate an adoption quest or decide to participate more in the lives of children in so many other enriching and beautiful ways. But what I wish for is that every queer person on this journey, I hope that you can take comfort in the community of our stories. I hope that we can remember to trust our queer magic: Radical love is not bound by genetic lineage or bodies,

> Western medicine, or registration forms. Our love is dancing
> toward liberation. Our queerness will be and is already
> enough to nourish and carry us through every twist and
> letdown. We already know how to make family outside the
> lines. —Nikiko Masumoto

If you are in the process of navigating the deeply challenging process of miscarriage and infertility, you are not alone. There are other queer people and hopeful solo parents in our communities grappling with similar feelings and experiences. Although this doesn't make it any easier, we do hope that it helps you feel less isolated. Lean into your people, and be with your feelings. We promise—you will get through this.

CHAPTER 9

Protecting Our Families: Legal Considerations and Building Community Resilience

Okay, now that we've talked about all the logistics of *how* to build our families, let's zoom out a bit and think about how we can protect our families. This chapter will focus on legal considerations for LGBTQ+ and solo parent families as well as poly families. We will also discuss other ways of protecting our families—by building community resilience and support.

In preparation for writing this chapter, we spoke with family lawyers Ora Prochovnik and Rebecca Levin Nayak, who have spent their careers working for legal recognition and protection of LGBTQ+ families. Ora says, "One of my favorite things about queer family law is that we can use the law creatively, but also creatively define what is family." While the legal landscape is different all over the country, and varies state by state, people have always and will continue to creatively find ways to legally protect our families.

In the following pages, we will go through the different legal considerations of protecting our families, including severing a known donor's rights after the birth of a child, second parent adoption, surrogacy arrangements, step-parent adoption, and recommended legal protections specific for solo parents. We will also explore the complex world of legal protection for polyamorous families.

We are not lawyers, and this chapter is meant only as an introduction to the concepts and questions you need to be familiar with in order to legally protect your family. The information in this section will be particularly US-focused, and there are big differences in protections in every state in the US—so we strongly recommend that you speak with an expert about family law where you live.

First Things First—Acknowledging the Oppression

To be honest, we feel resentful that we even need to write this section of the book. We know that most heterosexual couples, even if they are unmarried, never need to think about these extra legal protections for their families. The fact that we as LGBTQ+ and solo parents need to think, plan for, and pay to legally protect our families is deeply based in homophobia, cis-heterosexism, and our legal system's profound attachment to the institution of heterosexual marriage.

> I f*cking hated that I needed to adopt my own child. It just pissed me off that although I was this baby's baba, had wanted them, had helped my wife conceive them, had changed so many diapers…but I wasn't considered their legal parent. It was a reminder of all the oppression queer families still face in this world. But it also helped me appreciate my community that never once questioned me as my child's true parent. —Jules

Even though these legal considerations are based in oppression, we believe that it is important to protect our families in this way so we don't experience greater systemic harm. Our goal is to empower our readers (you!) to know your next steps so you and your children, partners, and donors will be taken care of. Let's start with talking about known donors.

Known Donor 101

In some states, knowing your sperm donor personally means that they have, by default, parental rights following the birth of the child. These rights include custody, decision making, and the responsibility of child support. Some states see the known donor contract as legally binding—but other states do not offer these protections.

As we mentioned in chapter 2, when people donate sperm or eggs to a bank, they already complete the legal process of rescinding their parenting rights. If a donor is known by a family, especially if the process of donation and conception involves a doctor or midwife, the paperwork you fill out stating the intended relationship and assisted insemination or IVF can create some clarity in legal proceedings after the child is born.

If you are in a partnership where both parents are not genetically related to the child, are using a traditional surrogate, or are building your family with reciprocal IVF, the next legal step is to confirm parenting rights and sever the donor's rights after birth through adoption. If you used a known donor, in some states your donor will also fill out paperwork to terminate their parental rights as part of the adoption process. By filing this paperwork, they legally and permanently rescind the parenting rights assigned to them because of the genetic relationship.

For solo parents who used a known donor, the process is less straightforward. Some states have laws regarding parentage with assisted reproductive technologies, and others do not. Get to know the laws in your state to learn if utilizing a doctor or midwife for inseminations creates helpful legal barriers between you and your donor. Rebecca Levin Nayak recommends utilizing and notarizing a known donor agreement prior to conception. Additionally, some states may allow you to pursue a pre-birth order declaring that you are a single parent, protecting you from future issues with not having two parents on the birth certificate.

What Is the Deal with Adopting Your Own Kid?

Confirmatory adoption is the process of a person who has always been a child's parent but is not genetically related to them going through a legal adoption. There are a few terms that are used to describe the adoption process. The most common are: *second parent adoption*, which means the non-genetic parent pursuing adoption is not married to the biological parent of the baby, and *step-parent adoption*, which includes both non-gestational parents who are married to the biological parent of the baby at the time of birth and parents who marry after the birth of a child and are legally adopting their stepchild. States with the most progressive assisted reproduction laws have a *confirmatory adoption* process.

Marea went through the process of step-parent adoption when legally adopting her two older kids, because she and her wife weren't married when they were born. Marea and her wife did get married before Marea gave birth to their third child, which, because they live in California, meant that they only needed to go through the confirmatory adoption process.

The differences among these types of adoption have to do with what steps must be taken to legally adopt the child, and each state will vary to some degree with requirements. For example, in Pennsylvania a step-parent adoption process includes child abuse clearances and a criminal records check for the past five years, an affidavit from the sperm bank and healthcare provider explaining how the insemination happened, and filing paperwork with the county clerk's office, all of which culminates in a court case when a judge pronounces your family legally bound. With a known donor, a petition to confirm the consent of the donor and description of how inseminations were performed is also provided. If the parents are not married, a second parent adoption often requires a home study by a social worker, but that is county-dependent.

In states that Ora calls "friendly jurisdictions" for LGBTQ+ and other nontraditional families, confirmatory adoptions are a lot simpler, typically not requiring home study, background checks, or even court dates. In certain states, like California, parents don't need to be legally married in order to complete a confirmatory adoption, but it does simplify the process if they are legally married before the birth of the child.

For Marea in California, the step-parent adoption process involved consulting with a lawyer, having a social worker assigned to her case (with whom she met only once), and finally having a judge declare her an adoptive parent. The process took about twenty-four months but was complicated by the COVID-19 pandemic. Meanwhile Marea's and her partner's confirmatory adoption involved simply filing some paperwork in the court, which took about ten months to process.

HOW TO FIND A LAWYER SPECIALIZING IN LGBTQ+ FAMILY LAW

It's really powerful to have a lawyer that gets you and that you trust. The legal system sucks, and to have someone who gets you makes a huge difference.
—Sarah, who parents with her wife and girlfriend

The LGBTQ+ Bar has a family law institute and directory of LGBTQ+ family lawyers to help you find an affirming lawyer in your state. You can learn more at www.lgbtqbar.org. Many of these lawyers support solo parent families as well.

Whatever your situation, we recommend consulting with a family lawyer familiar with the laws in your area to determine which path makes the most sense for your family. At the time of this writing, fees for filing for adoption on your own range from $200 to $2,000, depending on whether or not the court charges for visits from the social worker. With the support of a family lawyer, you can expect to add about $1,000 to $2,000 more to that initial fee.[1]

WHAT IF BOTH MY PARTNER'S AND MY NAMES ARE ON THE BIRTH CERTIFICATE? DO WE STILL NEED TO DO CONFIRMATORY ADOPTION?

Many states allow both parents in a queer relationship and married to put their names on the birth certificate, but only some see this as legal proof of parenthood in the state. Even if both parents' names are on the birth certificate, this does *not* provide legal parenting protection in all fifty states. The only way to protect yours and a non-gestational partner's parenting rights nationwide is confirmatory adoption.

While this is clearly based in heterosexism and homophobia, we do believe that it's important for LGBTQ+ parents to legally adopt their children to minimize the potential of legal discrimination in the future with travel, medical decision-making, or divorce.

Polyamory and Legal Family-Formation Options

At the time of this writing, there are no clear legal protections for poly families that hold across all fifty states. The case of Ian Jenkins and his partners Alan and Jeremy in California in 2017 was the first instance where a poly family all gained parenting rights, and there are a handful of states that allow additional parents through step-parent adoption. Ora has completed third and fourth parent adoptions in the state of California, but these don't necessarily hold up in courts in other states.

Poly families need to get extra creative in the process of trying to legally protect their families. There are mechanisms like wills, guardianship, and in loco parentis (a document stating rights that one can have in place of a parent) that can allow for parenting succession in the case of death. An example of creative protections may include filing custody arrangement documents with the courts after birth to memorialize your parenting intentions for your family and arrange for the in loco parentis parent to have custodial rights. We recommend talking to a lawyer in your state to learn what protections may be available for you in your particular poly family constellation.

> We did trusts, and then we had ten thousand attorneys to draft our embryo creation and surrogacy docs, and then a parenting agreement, and a legal battle to become the first poly family ever awarded parentage on a birth certificate! —Ian Jenkins, author of *Three Dads and a Baby*

Surrogacy

Before conception plans are put into motion, surrogacy starts with a lawyer and a contract to protect the intended parents' and surrogate's rights. Typically, with gestational surrogates, lawyers can write up the initial contracts between intended parents and surrogates outlining every expectation and can also assist with overseeing the execution of the pre-birth order that places the intended parents on the birth certificate before birth. Intended parents are responsible for all legal fees and will typically cover legal representation for their surrogate as well.

With traditional surrogacy, the legal process follows the adoption framework. Rebecca recommends writing up initial contracts before conception; after the baby is born, the parent who provided sperm is initially on the birth certificate, and the second intended parent pursues second parent or confirmatory adoption. During the process of second parent adoption the traditional surrogate surrenders their parenting rights, and the other intended parent legally adopts the child.

Details in the legal contract will depend very much on the state where the surrogate gives birth. Some places, like California, offer very clear protections for both surrogates and intended parents. Others, like New York, have actually outlawed surrogacy. For families interested in surrogacy that live in a state where it is illegal, many of them find surrogates who live in different states with friendlier laws. Some just accept the legal risks and do it anyway. The costs of legal services for surrogacy at the time of this writing range from $2,500 to $5,000 for initial contracts, $2,500 to $3,500 for pre-birth orders, and similar second parent adoption costs of $2,000 to $3,500 with lawyers.

Creative Family Connections developed a US Surrogacy Map to help consumers better understand surrogacy laws in every state to assist with decision-making, which you can find on their website at www.creativefamilyconnections.com/us-surrogacy-law-map.

Having to jump through legal hoops to legitimize our families in the eyes of the law is, unfortunately, a form of discrimination our families still have to deal with. But even though this conversation about legal protections for our families is intense, our families are worth all this emotional energy, all this time and money, all the research, logistics, and planning. And of course, we know that laws don't legitimize family—love and commitment do.

Protecting Ourselves Beyond the Law: How Building Community Resilience Supports Our Families

We know that legal forms are not the only way to protect our families. While there are huge benefits to us and our children when we use the law to support our families, there are also other, more intangible ways of protecting our family structures and values. In this section of the book, we explore how to create support systems through building resilience in our extended families and communities.

How to Build Resilience in Ourselves—Normalizing Our Experiences

Building resilience and tapping into our support systems starts with ourselves. Sometimes the heteropatriarchal model of family— heterosexual, married, thin, white, extremely gendered—can feel stifling. Yet families who don't fit into this model—queer families, single-parent families, poly families, blended families, and divorced families—have always existed. Although we are in good, growing company, our families are still considered radical in mainstream society.

Part of the reason we wrote this book is to help people feel less alone in their family-building choices. If nothing else, we hope you believe that your family is valid, beautiful, important, and that there are thousands of other families out there like yours. In twenty years, we hope that the information presented in this book is common knowledge. That young queer people easily see their parenting pathways reflected in the families of their friends and in media, that solo parenting is celebrated and normalized, and that all parents have more support in creating and raising children.

For now, we are all participating in changing this paradigm. We got this. We see you. It's not easy, but your choice of creating family

outside the heterosexual nuclear family model is radical and important. We stand on the shoulders of our queer ancestors in paving the
way for future generations of cultural visionaries.

When we normalize our experiences of family, we draw from
wells of support that maybe we didn't even know we needed. We
spoke a little in chapter 5 about how, if you're a trans pregnant person, it can be very powerful to put up photos of other trans people
who were pregnant and had babies, even if you don't know them.
Because of the oppressions that our families still face, we need to
draw support from our extended communities. It may sound silly to
print out photos from the internet, but we promise, visual representation matters immensely.

Another way we can support ourselves is through having books
that reflect our unique family structures. In the appendix, we offer
some book recommendations that reflect all different kinds of families. Being able to read to our children stories about families like ours
can be a balm to the heart when so much of our outside world doesn't
validate our family structure.

Throughout this whole journey, we encourage you to reach for
the feeling that you are connected to so many other people throughout your family-building process. Normalize your experience of
family building, and remember that you are in really good company.
LGBTQ+ parents, solo parents, and poly families have existed forever, and they sure as hell will never stop existing.

Oh, and be gentle with yourselves. Growing families and parenting with intention is intense work. Especially when we add the pain
of homophobia or the prejudice against unpartnered people, not to
mention the intersecting oppressions of racism, classism, ableism, et
cetera. You're contending with a lot. We hope you try, as much and as
often as you can, to treat yourself with kindness and tenderness and
so much compassion.

Building Resilience and Support Through Our Families of Origin and Extended Communities

Everyone has heard the old adage "It takes a village to raise a child." Unfortunately, in late-stage capitalism, our families are more isolated than they've ever been before. When we talk about building systems of support for our families, we are talking about actively countering the isolating force of capitalism that tries to separate us so we depend on things more than we depend on one another.

We know that for some people, building networks of support through their families of origin and extended communities can be more challenging than for others. While some of us are deeply connected to our communities, others may not be. Prospective solo parents may need to put extra focus on building their community support systems to help counter the isolation that is sometimes inherent to solo parenting.

In the following sections, we'll discuss navigating family-formation questions with your families of origin, which can be a complicated experience for many LGBTQ+ people and solo parents. We will also explore ways solo parents and poly families can plan for their parenting needs, offering hard-won community-sourced wisdom in how to build resilience both personally and within your communities.

Talking to Families of Origin About Our Family Formation Choices

If you're feeling confused, triggered, or unsure on how to approach talking to your family of origin about your family-building choices, you're in good company. No matter what kind of family you're building, for many of us, talking to our family of origin about our decisions is a nerve-racking and challenging task.

Planning for and having children tends to bring up memories from our own childhoods—the good, the bad, and the ugly—and can trigger hard feelings that we haven't yet healed. It can bring up deep feelings about how we feel we have (and have not) been accepted among our families of origin. Hopefully, these feelings can become good kindling for therapy sessions that can catapult our own healing and help us in turn become the parents we want to be.

People experience so many things when broaching these conversations with their families of origin—fear that their parents won't accept their child as their grandchild if they don't share DNA; concern that their families won't treat their partner as their child's other parent; fear that they will always experience judgment and misunderstanding from their families about choosing to become a solo parent; and so much more. In preparation for writing this section, we talked to dozens of people about how these conversations went for them. We also spoke with Hez Wollin, LCSW, a licensed social worker and queer parent, who helped us explore the nuances of these conversations from a mental health lens.

> I felt incredibly anxious about telling my family and my partner's family that I was pregnant. It mostly doesn't bother me to not be seen as nonbinary in day-to-day life, but the idea of being misgendered and called "mom" by my family was too much. —Til

For folks concerned that their pregnancy announcement will lead to misgendering, talk to partners, friends, and allied family members beforehand about how to announce the pregnancy and clearly communicate your parenting terms. Before initiating the conversation, make sure to arrange support for yourself among your community who see you as you are. You may choose to have this conversation at the same time as announcing your pregnancy or at another time in person or by email. Ray has had a few clients send queer parenting primers to their families, complete with their parenting terms and how they are navigating gender for the baby.

> I'll never forget when my mom asked incredulously if my same-sex partner would have legal rights to the child I was carrying, and I got to say "*Yes!* That is *exactly* what we want." It was so foreign to her, but she got the picture eventually. —Madelyn

When having these conversations, it can be helpful to have very clear boundaries, and to know when you are ready to end a conversation or if there are topics that are off-limits to discuss. Hez says, "You get to decide who you talk to and how much information you're willing to share. You are in charge." They encourage folks to think about what boundaries they want to have and to explore what is a hard boundary (something that you are unwilling to talk about with anyone) and what feels like a more flexible boundary. For example, someone may say, "I don't want to talk to my mom or dad about this, but I will talk to my siblings."

Hez also recommends knowing that you don't owe anyone any explanation about your choices. It's a good practice to get started on making those decisions about boundaries now, because once people become parents, they will be navigating this on a whole different level. As with everything, we recommend connecting with and leaning on your communities for support, as well as a therapist or other mental health professional.

> I asked my mom what questions she had about the donor we used to build our family, and I only answered the questions I was comfortable with. I've learned to have good boundaries with her questions (it helps our relationship

go better). Then, after talking for a while, I kindly asked her to let that curiosity with this unfamiliar process go, and just accept our family as our family. We were clear up front that terms like *dad* or *father* were not acceptable to us, and only the word *donor* should be used. Setting this boundary firmly early on proved helpful for us. —Alex

Of course, some people have families of origin who just won't get on board with their family-building choices because of deep-seated religious homophobia or other oppressive ideas about people and families. For folks in this situation, we encourage you to feel whatever comes up in processing building your own family while being unwelcomed by the one that you come from.

For everybody, but particularly those without families of origin to connect with, it's extra important to get extended communities on board for supporting the parenting process. As people forming families in creative and radical ways, that doesn't just stop with us. By nurturing our extended communities in relation to the families we are creating, we develop support systems for our children and ourselves that offer us the resilience and support we need and deserve.

We want to highlight that calling on our community support systems is *especially* important during the postpartum period. The time after giving birth or after your newborn is born (or even when adopting an older child) can be intensely destabilizing. Sleep deprivation, emotional overwhelm, and appointments and other logistical demands can make it impossible for new parents to feed themselves let alone take out the trash. Calling on our communities to support us during that time can make a profound difference to our and our child's experience of adjusting to the new family unit.

The Unique Joys and Challenges for Solo Parents by Choice

Our society doesn't know how to support parents, period. Parental leave is tenuous at best and nonexistent for many. Our friends, even though they mean well, are sometimes not prepared for what it takes to support someone with a new child. Society doesn't prepare us for the intense physical and emotional demands of parenthood, nor does capitalism encourage the kind of communal living and support that growing families actually need.

This lack of support can be especially glaring for solo parents. Choosing to have a child as a solo parent is amazing, and can also come with isolation. In this section, we want to lift up and honor the special aspects of solo parenting as well as offer community-sourced wisdom on how to navigate solo parenthood.

I chose to be a solo parent because I knew that for my future child to thrive, they needed me to be an empowered, joyful parent. I saw that I could be that, and it felt right to bring a child into my life. I felt inspired to decolonize what parenting meant to me and return to what I valued. To me, one solo parent was better than two parents that couldn't get along because that energy is all around the home. I had just learned that after exiting a long-term, unhealthy relationship.

As a single parent I loved that I led the vibration in our home. I appreciated the focus and present attention I was able to have with my children without distractions. Yes, my budget was tight, so we ate healthy simple foods and the Crock-Pot was pretty much always on. We listened to music and relaxed, picnicked at the park. We cuddled and took baths. On my days off work we took long naps together.

People seem surprised when I express that often our home life felt simple and easeful. I think it is not natural to have a baby in isolation, and I am extremely grateful to the friends who really came through and supported me through this phase, who celebrated my family with me. I chose to have two of my children as a single mama; now I am married and we've had another baby together. I like that having children wasn't something I had to put on the back burner until I found the right partner. —Andrea Ruizquez

We spoke to dozens of solo parents about what they love and what they struggle with regarding solo parenting in preparation for writing this section. What we learned is that so many solo parents love their lives! We also learned that it is *so* important to develop extended community support in the form of friends, neighbors, and other solo parents to cut through some of the isolation inherent in the day-to-day. One solo parent we talked to recommended having a list of three trusted people who agreed to be on your emergency team. This means that you can call them in the event of an emergency, and even if you don't end up calling, it makes a difference to know that you *can*. In the early postpartum period, have one trusted friend be your coordinator for meal trains and home support help.

How do you develop the community you need to parent? Some solo parents find their people through online solo parenting networks and local kid meetups, and others find them through participating in organizations that matter to them where they can meet people with shared interests. One parent recommended going to aqua aerobics to connect to seniors who may have more availability and excitement for spending time with babies. Nurturing your existing friendships, whether it's making time to go for a walk or remembering a friend's birthday, will also deepen relationships and mutual connection.

We also recommend trusting your instincts and not comparing yourself with anyone else—one of the many beautiful aspects of solo parenting is that you get to define what your life looks like with your child(ren). Don't compare yourselves with parent influencers or let anyone else tell you how much you can handle. That's one of the benefits of solo parenting—you get to be the one steering that ship.

> The thing I love most about being a solo parent is all the one-on-one bonding babe and I get. I feel like we are really in sync. I'm sure all parents feel like they know all their baby's special quirks and inside jokes, but as a solo parent you really do! —Flee, she/her, and Pickle, they/them

Another tip we heard from solo parents is to write affirmations. In hard moments, when the baby isn't sleeping or the fire alarm goes off after you accidentally burned dinner, it can be helpful to have affirmations up on the walls that are reminders to you that you are doing a good job. Affirmations as simple as "You got this" or "Breathe, this too shall pass" can go a long way. Try to give the same tenderness and love to yourself that you give to your child. Parenting can sometimes feel impossible, and it's so important to remember that we are always trying our best, even when it feels like we are falling short.

Lastly, prioritize self-care. This might seem impossible when you're home all day with a newborn, but finding moments to care for your body in the ways that felt good before becoming a parent will help you feel more like yourself. Self-care looks different with a child—maybe you paint your and your kid's toenails at home instead of going to a nail salon, or take nap time to soak in the bathtub, or do yoga next to your kid while they play. It may sound meager, but these little moments add up. Also, don't be afraid to lean on your support system or paid childcare, when you can, to get a break so you can care for yourself and enjoy parenting.

Poly Families

My platonic partner and I were both in committed romantic partnerships when we decided to start trying to get pregnant. While neither of our girlfriends would be acting as co-parent when the baby came, we wanted to make sure they didn't feel like we were doing something secretive, so inviting them over for the insemination felt like the least weird way to do a weird thing. My partner's girlfriend, my girlfriend, and I hung out in the living room and blasted cheesy '90s R&B while my partner collected a sample in the other room. I inseminated myself and we all watched *Rosemary's Baby* and ate popcorn after. It worked on the first round. —Ayden

In many ways, parenting in polyamorous relationships make so much sense: Parenting requires time, attention, and money, and having more than two parents in a family can provide extra resources that benefit the whole family immensely. If you are in a polyamorous family or are dreaming of creating one, you're not alone! It's wonderful to break out of the mold of the two-parent nuclear family and create a more expansive example of what a family can be.

If you're in polyamorous relationships, you know how important communication is. This becomes extra necessary when there is a child involved, and it's essential to be clear about everybody's roles in the child's life. Talk about one another's roles, including how decisions about this child's health and well-being will be made. Is it a democracy, or does one person have the final say? What if there are disagreements about where to send the kid to school or whether or not to give them sugar? Try having these conversations as early as possible to get a sense of one another's values around parenting, and practice working through hard conversations. Also, know that when a child comes into the world, it can change everything. Be open and willing to reevaluate previous agreements.

Changes in identity, relationship dynamics, sleep loss, and time add stress to any relationship. Plan for the transition ahead of time by identifying the resources each partner can utilize to care for themselves and one another in times of stress. Whether it is talking on the phone with a friend, going for a walk, having an hour in the morning to stretch, or utilizing a support group, each person will benefit from different types of self-care. In addition to planning for self-care, plan for connection.

Each individual relationship as well as the collective one needs time and care, and some partners will also have relationships outside their parenting polycule. It can take a few months to get into a groove with these new parenting roles and find time to show up for relationships. When time is scarce, seek smaller moments of nurturing connections. And just because there are three or more partners doesn't mean you can't hire a babysitter to go on a date! Caring for yourselves as adults and partners will allow you to parent better together.

When possible, explore legal protection for your family. True protections may not be possible, but there are often creative work-arounds to the laws in your state. Search for a family lawyer in your state who has experience working with polyamorous people to explore your options.

———

Whether it's through legal action or through building support systems within and around your family, we hope that what you take from this chapter (and this whole book) is that your family, whatever its structure, is precious and deserving of protection and support. There are so many ways to build resilience for our families, ourselves, our kids, and our extended communities.

Saying Goodbye (for Now)

Well, friends, we made it! Thank you for joining us on this journey—we know that the path to parenthood is a winding one, and we are glad to be able to keep you company. We also want to take another opportunity to shout out loud from the rooftops that WE LOVE YOUR FAMILY! We love and honor our communities—all the parents, the currently-in-existence and the soon-to-be-born children, and the much-needed transformation that we are bringing into the world by forming families in the ways that we do. Our families are essential gifts to the world.

We have thoroughly enjoyed the process of distilling what we know as midwives serving the LGBTQ+ and solo parent communities, and we truly hope that this book will support nascent families for years to come.

We also know that this book is just the beginning of our connection to you as a resource in growing your family. If you're not quite ready to say goodbye, you can connect with us through our website, www.babymakingforeverybody.com, where we will be collecting up-to-date information about support and resources for LGBTQ+ and solo parent families, as well as offering a blog featuring stories about LGBTQ+ and solo parent family formation. If you are interested in sharing your story with our extended community (and we really hope you are), you will find submission guidelines on our website. We also will continue to offer fertility care and home birth in our areas, and provide virtual fertility consultations to people wanting personalized guidance from us from afar.

Until next time, we wish you luck, joy, and as much ease as possible on your family-building journey. We are super stoked for you.

Acknowledgments

This book has been a labor of love that we could not have done without the support of our partners, friends, and community. Thank you to Brook Warner and her team for being our early book-doula and helping us clarify our goals and write our book proposal. Thank you to our agent Jessica Alvarez and our editor Hannah Robinson for believing the world needed this book. Thank you to our partners Asher and Andrea. Asher's love, experience, and fastidious Virgo editing contributed immensely to these pages, and Andrea's emotional support and sincere willingness to watch the kids so that Marea could write and edit made all of this possible.

We also want to name in gratitude all of the people who contributed their expertise and insight to these pages: Stephanie Hayes, Randall Wilson, Mykhia Odom, Laura Collins, JB Brown, Emily DeMartino, Camden Segal, Ellie Lobovits, Katy Giombilini, Rebecca Levin Nayak, Monica Martinez, Hez Wollin, Neill Sullivan, Ora Prochovnik, and River Nice. Thank you, Isabel Crosby, for formatting our citations for us. Thank you to everyone who submitted their story and followed our curveball of switching from an anthology to a guidebook. Thank you to the queer midwives that came before us that have made it possible for us to be out of the closet and earn a living. And thank you to our queer ancestors who paved the way, fought so hard, and loved so deeply so that we can be this out and proud about supporting more and more LGBTQ+ and solo parent families.

Appendix

Let Us Midwife You:
Resources for Family Formation

In the following pages we've collected resources with some of the nitty-gritty information you may still need to move forward in forming your family, including:

For the most up-to-date version of this information, and to download any of the templates, please visit our website: www.babymakingforeverybody.com.

Sample Letter to Ask for Sperm, Eggs, or a Uterus

Feeling awkward or unsure how to ask a potential donor if they're interested in sharing their sperm, eggs, or uterus with you? Here's an example of an email or letter you can edit to fit your needs and send to them.

Dear _____,

Thanks for taking the time to read this! We are A and B, a queer couple from _____. A is a mechanic and B is a teacher. We met five years ago while in school. We have been pursuing becoming parents for ___(amount of time)____, and are looking for a local sperm or egg donor to help us have a baby.

We would like to find a donor who is _____ (ethnicity, personality traits, et cetera)_____, nice, has no major family medical concerns, and is local to _____. Our ideal donor would understand that they have no parental rights over the child, and we are open to having a relationship with the donor that ranges from distant contact to family friend.

Being a sperm or egg donor would be a huge gift to our family. We would ask (and pay for) you to have an STI test and a sperm count before starting / all related medical costs for harvesting eggs. We also request to sign an agreement clarifying that we are the only intended parents. [For sperm donors only]: Donation would also involve on-call availability to provide a sperm sample once or twice a month.

If you're open to talking about becoming a donor for our family, please let us know when in the coming weeks we could take you out for coffee or ice cream or chat on Zoom.

Thank you for considering helping us become parents.

Sincerely,

A & B

Sample Known Donor Contract

We *strongly* recommend that anyone working with a known donor write a donor agreement before trying to conceive, whether with a lawyer or independently. Bear in mind that known donor agreements may or may not be legally enforceable in your state, but they can still serve as a tool for conversations about boundaries, expectations, and relationships during and after the donation process.

The LGBTQ+ Bar has a family law institute and directory of LGBTQ+ family lawyers to help you find an affirming lawyer in your state at www.lgbtqbar.org.

Sample Known Donor Contract (Sperm Donor Specific)

This   AGREEMENT   is   made   this   _____   day   of _____, 20___, by and between _____ _____, hereafter DONOR, and _____ _____, hereafter RECIPIENT, who may also be referred to herein as the parties.

NOW, THEREFORE, in consideration of the promises of each other, DONOR and RECIPIENT agree as follows:

1. Each clause of the AGREEMENT is separate and divisible from the others, and, should a court refuse to enforce one or more clauses of this AGREEMENT, the others are still valid and in full force.

2. DONOR has agreed to provide (her/their/his/name) semen to RECIPIENT for the purpose of artificial insemination.

3. In exchange, DONOR has received from RECIPIENT _____ (many people give a financial amount to signify the exchange).

4. Each party is a single person who has never married. (If either party is in a relationship or married, state that here.)

5. Each party acknowledges and agrees that, through the procedure of artificial insemination, the RECIPIENT is attempting to become pregnant. It is our intent that such inseminations shall continue until conception occurs.

6. Each party acknowledges and agrees that DONOR provided (her/their/his/name) semen for the purposes of said artificial insemination, and did so with the clear understanding that (she/they/he/name) would not demand, request, or compel any guardianship, custody, or visitation rights with any child born from the artificial insemination procedure. Further, DONOR acknowledges that (she/they/he/name) fully understands that (she/they/he/name) would have no parental rights whatsoever with said child.

7. Each party acknowledges and agrees that RECIPIENT has relinquished any and all rights that (she/they/he/name) might otherwise have to hold DONOR legally, financially, or emotionally responsible for any child that results from the artificial insemination procedure.

8. Each party acknowledges and agrees that the sole authority to name any child resulting from the artificial insemination procedure shall rest with RECIPIENT.

9. Each party acknowledges and agrees that there shall be no father named on the birth certificate of any child born from the artificial insemination procedure.

10. Each party relinquishes and releases any and all rights (she/they/he/name) may have to bring a suit to establish parenthood.

11. Each party covenants and agrees that, in light of the expectations of each party, as stated above, RECIPIENT shall have absolute authority and power to appoint a guardian for (her/their/his/name) child, and that the RECIPIENT and guardian may act with sole discretion as to all legal financial, medical, and emotional needs of said child without any involvement with or demands of authority from DONOR.

12. Each party covenants and agrees that the identity of the DONOR shall be made known to the child at a time and in a manner to be determined solely by the RECIPIENT. Each party reserves the right not to disclose (her/their/his/name) identity to any others, and RECIPIENT agrees not to disclose DONOR's identity to any specific persons upon (her/their/his/name) written request including full names. (If your donor has different desires around privacy, this paragraph should clarify that agreement.)

13. Each party acknowledges and agrees that the relinquishment of all rights, as stated above, is final and irrevocable. DONOR further understands that (her/their/his/name) waivers shall prohibit any action on (her/their/his/name) part for custody, guardianship, or visitation in any future situations, including the event of RECIPIENT's disability or death.

14. Each party acknowledges and understands that any future contact the DONOR may have with any child(ren) that result(s) from the artificial insemination procedure in no way alters the effect of this agreement. Any such contact will be at the discretion of the RECIPIENT and/or appointed guardian, and will be consistent with the intent of both parties to sever any and all parental rights and responsibilities of the DONOR.

15. Each party covenants and agrees that any dispute pertaining to this AGREEMENT that arises between them shall be submitted to binding arbitration according to the following procedures:

a. The request for arbitration may be made by either party and shall be in writing and delivered to the other party;

b. Pending the outcome of arbitration, there shall be no change made in the language of this AGREEMENT;

c. The arbitration panel that will resolve any disputes regarding this AGREEMENT shall consist of three persons: one person chosen by DONOR, one person chosen by RECIPIENT, and one person chosen by the other two panel members;

d. Within fourteen calendar days following the written arbitration request, the arbitrators shall be chosen;

e. Within fourteen days following the selection of all members of the arbitration panel, the panel will hear the dispute between parties;

f. Within seven days subsequent to the hearing, the arbitration panel will make a decision and communicate it in writing to each party.

16. Each party acknowledges and understands that there are legal questions raised by the issues involved in this AGREEMENT that have not been settled by statute or prior court decisions. Notwithstanding the knowledge that certain of the clauses stated herein may not be enforced in a court of law, the parties choose to enter into this AGREEMENT and clarify their intent that existed at the time the artificial insemination procedure was implemented by them.

17. Each party acknowledges and agrees that (she/they/he/name) signed this AGREEMENT voluntarily and freely, of (her/their/his/name) own choice, without any duress of any kind whatsoever. It is further acknowledged that each party has been advised to secure the advice and consent of an attorney of (her/their/his/name) own choosing, and that each party understands the meaning and significance of each provision of this AGREEMENT.

18. Each party acknowledges and agrees that any changes made in the terms and conditions of the AGREEMENT shall be made in writing and signed by both parties.

19. This AGREEMENT contains the entire understanding of the parties. There are no promises, understandings, agreements, or representations between the parties other than those expressly stated in this AGREEMENT.

IN WITNESS WHEREOF, the parties hereto have executed this AGREEMENT, in the city of _____ _____, and the state of _____, on the day and year first above written.

Donor Signature Donor Name (Print): _____

Recipient Signature Recipient Name (Print): _____

Fertility Tracker Template

NAME _____   AGE _____   MONTH _____

CYCLE DAY	1	2	3	4	5	6	7	8	9	10	11	12	13	14	15	16	17
DATE																	

| BASAL BODY TEMPERATURE (F) | 99 9 8 7 6 5 4 3 2 1 98 9 8 7 6 5 4 3 2 1 97 9 | 99 9 8 7 6 5 4 3 2 1 98 9 8 7 6 5 4 3 2 1 97 9 | 99 9 8 7 6 5 4 3 2 1 98 9 8 7 6 5 4 3 2 1 97 9 | 99 9 8 7 6 5 4 3 2 1 98 9 8 7 6 5 4 3 2 1 97 9 | 99 9 8 7 6 5 4 3 2 1 98 9 8 7 6 5 4 3 2 1 97 9 | 99 9 8 7 6 5 4 3 2 1 98 9 8 7 6 5 4 3 2 1 97 9 | 99 9 8 7 6 5 4 3 2 1 98 9 8 7 6 5 4 3 2 1 97 9 | 99 9 8 7 6 5 4 3 2 1 98 9 8 7 6 5 4 3 2 1 97 9 | 99 9 8 7 6 5 4 3 2 1 98 9 8 7 6 5 4 3 2 1 97 9 | 99 9 8 7 6 5 4 3 2 1 98 9 8 7 6 5 4 3 2 1 97 9 | 99 9 8 7 6 5 4 3 2 1 98 9 8 7 6 5 4 3 2 1 97 9 | 99 9 8 7 6 5 4 3 2 1 98 9 8 7 6 5 4 3 2 1 97 9 | 99 9 8 7 6 5 4 3 2 1 98 9 8 7 6 5 4 3 2 1 97 9 | 99 9 8 7 6 5 4 3 2 1 98 9 8 7 6 5 4 3 2 1 97 9 | 99 9 8 7 6 5 4 3 2 1 98 9 8 7 6 5 4 3 2 1 97 9 | 99 9 8 7 6 5 4 3 2 1 98 9 8 7 6 5 4 3 2 1 97 9 | 99 9 8 7 6 5 4 3 2 1 98 9 8 7 6 5 4 3 2 1 97 9 |

CERVICAL FLUID																	
CERVICAL POSITION																	
CERVICAL OPENNESS																	

| OPK | | | | | | | | | | | | | | | | | |

| INSEMINATION? | | | | | | | | | | | | | | | | | |

| NOTES | | | | | | | | | | | | | | | | | |

18	19	20	21	22	23	24	25	26	27	28	29	30	31	32	33	34	35	36	37	38	39	40
99	99	99	99	99	99	99	99	99	99	99	99	99	99	99	99	99	99	99	99	99	99	99
9	9	9	9	9	9	9	9	9	9	9	9	9	9	9	9	9	9	9	9	9	9	9
8	8	8	8	8	8	8	8	8	8	8	8	8	8	8	8	8	8	8	8	8	8	8
7	7	7	7	7	7	7	7	7	7	7	7	7	7	7	7	7	7	7	7	7	7	7
6	6	6	6	6	6	6	6	6	6	6	6	6	6	6	6	6	6	6	6	6	6	6
5	5	5	5	5	5	5	5	5	5	5	5	5	5	5	5	5	5	5	5	5	5	5
4	4	4	4	4	4	4	4	4	4	4	4	4	4	4	4	4	4	4	4	4	4	4
3	3	3	3	3	3	3	3	3	3	3	3	3	3	3	3	3	3	3	3	3	3	3
2	2	2	2	2	2	2	2	2	2	2	2	2	2	2	2	2	2	2	2	2	2	2
1	1	1	1	1	1	1	1	1	1	1	1	1	1	1	1	1	1	1	1	1	1	1
98	98	98	98	98	98	98	98	98	98	98	98	98	98	98	98	98	98	98	98	98	98	98
9	9	9	9	9	9	9	9	9	9	9	9	9	9	9	9	9	9	9	9	9	9	9
8	8	8	8	8	8	8	8	8	8	8	8	8	8	8	8	8	8	8	8	8	8	8
7	7	7	7	7	7	7	7	7	7	7	7	7	7	7	7	7	7	7	7	7	7	7
6	6	6	6	6	6	6	6	6	6	6	6	6	6	6	6	6	6	6	6	6	6	6
5	5	5	5	5	5	5	5	5	5	5	5	5	5	5	5	5	5	5	5	5	5	5
4	4	4	4	4	4	4	4	4	4	4	4	4	4	4	4	4	4	4	4	4	4	4
3	3	3	3	3	3	3	3	3	3	3	3	3	3	3	3	3	3	3	3	3	3	3
2	2	2	2	2	2	2	2	2	2	2	2	2	2	2	2	2	2	2	2	2	2	2
1	1	1	1	1	1	1	1	1	1	1	1	1	1	1	1	1	1	1	1	1	1	1
97	97	97	97	97	97	97	97	97	97	97	97	97	97	97	97	97	97	97	97	97	97	97
9	9	9	9	9	9	9	9	9	9	9	9	9	9	9	9	9	9	9	9	9	9	9

Lifestyle Interventions to Promote Fertility

Universal Interventions

- Eat whole foods.
- Maintain blood sugar with regular protein intake.
- Try acupuncture.
- Support optimal liver filtration by minimizing alcohol, caffeine, drugs.
- Stop smoking.
- Stay hydrated.
- Exercise regularly, not too intensely.
- Prioritize sleep.
- Manage stress.

Fertility Support Specific for People with Testes

Nutrition and Supplements

- Cruciferous vegetables (broccoli, kale, cabbage), vegetables with beta-carotene (carrots) and lycopene (tomatoes).[1]

Antioxidants

Our favorites on these lists are marked with a star.

- N-acetyl-cysteine: 600 mg/day*
- CoQ10: 400mg/day*
- L-carnitine: 2–3g/day
- Acetyl-L-carnitine: 3g/day
- Glutathione: 600mg/day
- Astaxanthin: 16mg/day
- Lycopene: 4–8mg/day*

Herbs

- Ashwagandha: 675mg/day*
- Tribulus: 250mg/day
- Maca: 1500–3000mg/day

Vitamins

- Vitamin C + vitamin E: 1g/day
- Folic acid: 5mg/day*
- Zinc: 66mg/day*
- Selenium: 100mg/day

Lifestyle Interventions

- Avoid human-made estrogens.
- Avoid hot tubs.
- Promote blood flow to testicles.

Fertility Support Specific for People with Uteruses

Nutrition and Supplements

- Prenatal or multivitamin with 400mcg folate, not folic acid
- Maca: 1000–3000mg/day[2]
- Vitex: 4 droppers full of tincture 3x/day
- CoQ10: 200mg/day
- Vitamin D: 2000 IU/day
- Omega-3: 1500 IU/day

Lifestyle Interventions

- Eat whole foods, focusing on healthy fats, high fiber, and good sources of protein with every meal.
- Eat regularly and prioritize a big breakfast.
- Try acupuncture.

- Avoid or minimize alcohol, cigarettes, energy drinks, very processed foods, and caffeine consumption.
- Stay hydrated.
- Exercise regularly, but not too intensely.

Finding an Affirming Provider

When Ray walked into Callen Lorde, an LGBTQ Health Center, at age twenty-one, it was the first time they ever experienced queer-competent, respectful healthcare. It was life changing to work with a provider who could actually answer their health questions in a kind, respectful manner. Now as midwives, we have the privilege of providing affirming healthcare experiences to others. We want everyone reading this book to have queer- and solo-parent-affirming care while going through the hugeness of growing your family.

So how do you find your affirming provider? Start with community recommendations, LGBTQ+ health centers, and referrals from a provider whom you currently like and trust. The Family Equality Council has a directory of providers who have taken their competency training, and *Psychology Today* and the LGBTQ Bar Association have directories of LGBTQ practitioners in every state. Health at Every Size has directories of size-affirming providers, and the Queer Doula Network is a national database of queer doulas.

Next, did you know you can interview and screen providers? You can either ask to have some questions answered by the provider on the phone before establishing care; ask if a clinic or midwife does complimentary consultations to see if you're a good fit; or, if cost and insurance allow, schedule an intake appointment and interview your provider before starting your health history, beginning any clinical assessment, or removing any clothing.

Here are some sample questions to ask a provider:
- How many LGBTQ+ people have you cared for?
- What percentage of your practice is currently LGBTQ+?
- What percentage of your practice is solo parents?
- How does your care differ when working with solo parents / LGBTQ+ people? How is it the same?
- Are your intake forms and handouts inclusive of solo parents / LGBTQ+ people?
- Have your front desk staff, nurses, and other people participating in my care received training in affirming language and working with solo parents / LGBTQ+ people?
- Have you participated in continuing education around caring for LGBTQ+ families? How much, and how has it changed how you care for patients?
- What is your practice's experience with insurance billing advocacy for solo parents / LGBTQ+ people, since we often do not meet infertility criteria? Does your billing department provide advocacy or accommodations and assistance due to discrimination solo parents / LGBTQ+ people face?

Notice the language the provider and front desk staff use—does it make you feel comfortable, or not?

What if there isn't an affirming provider in your area? Plan for advocacy by bringing a trusted friend, partner, or doula to your visit. Outline your needs, priorities, and questions before your appointment and write them down. Stay clothed until all your questions are answered, ask for clarification if inappropriate questions are asked, and don't answer anything you don't want to. If you don't feel safe, you can decline being touched and leave, or you can choose to proceed with clinical care and process the experience afterward. If you have feedback for how the provider or office could do a better job with your care, put it in writing and submit it.

The medical system can create a perceived power imbalance that is very unequal and hierarchical, and negative experiences in healthcare often reinforce that. It can sometimes take years to learn to challenge this dynamic and internalize the belief that you are an equal, and a consumer who is hiring a provider to meet a specific need instead of a sick person needing to be treated. Practice saying no in small ways so you feel more confident when you say yes.

As we said earlier, we are *huge* proponents of shifting power in healthcare dynamics. Some of the ways Ray does this for themself include:

- Refusing to be weighed or have a weight charted.
- Choosing providers who are peers, and choosing nurse practitioners (NPs) or physician assistants (PAs) over medical doctors (MDs).
- Starting care with a telehealth appointment.
- Coming into the appointment with questions and concerns to be addressed written out.
- Declining any clinical exam (including blood pressure) until all their questions have been answered to their satisfaction.
- Always wearing their own clothes.
- Discussing consent and removal of consent prior to any internal exams, and inserting the speculum themself.
- Providing direct feedback in the moment when a provider says or does something that doesn't feel good for them or if their paperwork was not inclusive.

Ray is a white healthcare provider, so the way she can advocate assertively in healthcare spaces is different from people experiencing more systemic harm. You don't have to adopt Ray's style of advocacy, but we hope some of these ideas might inspire some of the ways you communicate and seek care. You deserve to have a provider that sees you, respects you, and can provide holistic care for your whole family.

Understanding Fertility Research: How to Google and Get (Good) Information

It can be really difficult to parse information about fertility options, success rates, and how information applies to your body. There are two reasons for this.

First, most information about fertility options exist on the websites of fertility clinics, which are trying to sell you their services. Unfortunately, it's not uncommon for clinics to manipulate their data to claim higher success rates for IUI and IVF than are found in medical studies. This is done by excluding certain information from a study, BMI cutoffs, or not offering IVF to people over a certain age without donor eggs. In fact, data manipulation became so rampant that the Centers for Disease Control (CDC) now requires fertility clinics to report their data to a national database, where consumers can view actual rates for the clinics they are interested in.

When you're searching online articles that address your questions about fertility or providers, the first thing to check is who owns the website. Most articles about fertility options and intervention are on fertility clinic websites. These articles can be informative and offer a wealth of information to assist you in family planning; however, we encourage you to read with a critical eye—especially on pregnancy success rates. Additionally, many LGBTQ+-specific fertility websites are owned by fertility clinics, and other information about fertility in our community comes from sponsored posts by fertility clinics.

Here are three reputable sources we refer to that accurately report success rates with different fertility procedures:

- https://www.reproductivefacts.org/ (from the Society for Assisted Reproductive Medicine)
- https://www.fertilityiq.com (developed as an evidenced-based resource by a couple after going through a difficult experience with infertility clinics)
- https://www.cdc.gov/art/artdata/index.html (the CDC ART Success Rate database for all fertility clinics as well as a tool for predicting IVF success)

The second reason, as we talked about in chapter 8, is that most of the data we have on infertility is based on infertile, cisgender heterosexual couples needing infertility treatment. Research with lesbian couples, transgender individuals, and single people seeking fertility care does exist, but the data about how our bodies respond to fertility interventions is not of the same standard as what mainstream infertility care is based on. As you research your options online, just keep in mind that the system and the information guiding this system are not built for us.

Financing

There are grants available for people experiencing infertility or needing financial help for assisted reproductive technologies or adoption. Family Equality and Connecting Rainbows maintain ongoing lists where folks can apply for funds. Additionally, some fertility clinics have funds and grants to cover portions of treatment. We've included a list below, as well as on our website.

- AGC Scholarship Foundation
- BabyQuest Foundation
- The Family Formation Charitable Trust
- Queer Family Planning Project
- American Academy of Adoption Attorneys' Family Formation Charitable Trust
- Carolina Conceptions
- EMD Serrono Compassionate Care
- Gift of Adoption Fund
- Gift of Parenthood
- Hasidah
- Helpusadopt.org
- Journey to Parenthood
- Men Having Babies—Gay Parenting Assistance Program
- National Adoption Foundation Financial Program
- Reunite Assist
- Starfish Infertility Foundation
- The Hope for Fertility National Grant

It is also possible to put some of your costs—say, lawyer fees for second parent adoption—on a baby registry.

ACCESSING RESOURCES SECONDHAND

A wealth of supplies for baby making and pregnancy (ovulation predictor kits, books, syringes) already exists within our community, as do baby supplies. Join your local queer exchange and LGBTQ+ parenting groups, and also go to local secondhand stores or Craigslist.

Finding Community

We know we keep saying this, but really, community is so important. We have a revolving list of support groups on our website, but here are some of the city and state LGBTQ+ organizations and family pride groups you may find community in.

If your local LGBTQ+ center does not have a prospective parents group, reach out and request one! Forty-eight to fifty-three percent of LGBTQ+ millennials want to parent, so you are not alone in your search for community.[3] PFLAG—Parents, Family, and Friends of Lesbian and Gays—is the largest LGBTQ family organization in the US, and they have chapters in almost every area of the country. Go to https://pflag.org to find local community.

Alabama

Magic City Parents: https://www.magiccityparents.com/
Magic City Acceptance Center: https://www.MagicCity
   AcceptanceCenter.org

Alaska

Identity, Inc. (Gay & Lesbian Community Center of Anchorage):
   www.identityinc.org

Arizona

Bullhead City LGBTQ Pride Center: https://www.lgbtqaware
   nessofaz.com
Transspectrum of Arizona: https://tsaz.org
Phoenix Pride Center: http://phoenixpridelgbtcenter.org

Arkansas

Northwest Arkansas Equality: https://www.nwaequality.org

California

Sacramento Gay Dads: https://www.meetup.com/Sacramento DadsGroup/

Sacramento Area Rainbow Families: https://www.facebook .com/groups/434008199969774/about/

Billy DeFrank LGBTQ Community Center: https://www .defrankcenter.org

Stonewall Alliance Center of Chico: http://www.stonewallchico .org/

Rainbow Community Center of Contra Costa County: http:// www.rainbowcc.org/

The Diversity Center: http://www.diversitycenter.org/

Pacific Pride Foundation—North County: http://www.pacific pridefoundation.org/

Spectrum: http://www.spectrummarin.org/

San Francisco LGBT Community Center: http://www.sfcenter.org/

LGBTQ Center OC: https://www.lgbtqcenteroc.org

Pacific Center: https://www.pacificcenter.org

Yolo Rainbow Families: https://www.facebook.com/yolo rainbowfamilies/

LGBTQ Perinatal Welllness Center: https://www.LGBTQ PerinatalWellnessCenter.com

Our Family Coalition: https://www.ourfamily.org

Pop Luck Club: http://www.popluckclub.org

LA Genderqueer Parenting: https://www.facebook.com/LAGQ Parenting/

Center Long Beach Queer Parenting Group: https://www .centerlb.org/groups/

Creating Kin Collective: https://www.sdfamilywellness.com

San Diego Gay Dads: https://www.facebook.com/groups /291115988050709/about/

The San Diego LGBT Center: https://thecentersd.org/programs/family-services/

Colorado

LGBTQ Family Program Denver: https://lgbtqcolorado.org/programs/lgbtq-family/

Queer and Trans Parents in Boulder: https://www.boulderlgbtqiaparents.com

Colorado Lesbian Moms: https://www.facebook.com/groups/812255972474456/about/

Connecticut

New Haven Gay and Lesbian Community Center: https://www.newhavenpridecenter.org

Delaware

Delaware Pride: http://www.delawarepride.org

Florida

Florida LGBT Foster and Adoptive Parent Association: https://m.facebook.com/groups/386909214830202/

Jacksonville LGBT Families / Parenting with Pride North Florida: jacksonvillelgbtfamilies@gmail.com or https://www.facebook.com/ParentingwithPrideNorthFlorida/

LGBTQ+ Families of Central Florida: https://m.facebook.com/groups/lgbtqparentsofcentralflorida/

Metro Wellness & Community Centers: https://www.metrotampabay.org/

South Florida Family Pride, Inc.: https://www.facebook.com/SouthFloridaFamilyPride/

Pridelines Miami LGBTQ Center: https://pridelines.org/#

The Center Orlando: https://thecenterorlando.org

The Gay and Lesbian Community Center of South Florida: https://www.compassglcc.com

The Pride Center at Equality Park: https://www.pride centerflorida.org/

Georgia

Two Mommies Atlanta: https://www.facebook.com/groups/two mommiesatlanta/about/

Atlanta Pride: https://www.atlantapride.org

Hawaii

Hawaii LGBT Legacy Foundation: http:// hawaiilgbtlegacyfoundation.com/

Idaho

The Community Center: www.tccidaho.org/

Illinois

Affinity 95: https://www.affinity95.org

Center on Halsted: https://www.centeronhalsted.org

Indiana

Pride Lafayette: http://www.pridelafayette.org

Indy Pride: https://indypride.org

Iowa

Adair Co GLBT Resource Center: http://www.adaircoglbt resourcecenter.com

Kansas

The Center of Wichita: http://www.thecenterofwichita.org/

Modern Family Alliance: https://modernfamilyalliance.word press.com/

Kentucky

Gay & Lesbian Services Organization & Pride Center of the
Bluegrass: www.glso.org

Louisiana

NOLA Gay Families: https://m.facebook.com/groups
/222525154800016/

LGBT Community Center of New Orleans: https://
lgbtccneworleans.org

Maine

Out Maine: https://outmaine.org

Maryland

The GLBT Community Center of Baltimore: www.glccb.org/

Massachusetts

Keshet Families with Young Children: https://www.kesheton
line.org

Rainbow Families of Woburn: https://www.facebook.com
/groups/rainbowfamilieswoburn/about/

Gay Fathers of Greater Boston: https://www.gayfathersboston.org

Fenway Health LGBTQIA+ Family and Parenting Services:
https://fenwayhealth.org/care/wellness-resources
/lgbtqia-family-services/

South Coast LGBTQ Network: https://www.sclgbtqnetwork.org

Michigan

LGBTQ+ Parents of Ann Arbor / Ypsilanti: https://m.facebook
.com/groups/AnnArborYpsiLGBTQFamilies/

Lesbian Moms' Network: www.lmnetwork.org

Affirmations: www.goaffirmations.org/

Minnesota

Twin Cities Pride: https://www.tcpride.org

Twin Cities Queer Families: https://www.facebook.com/groups
/233662700049154/

Gay and Bi Fathers Support Group: https://www.meetup.com
/FathersGroup/?_cookie-check=CR4Ii8Nnnf2Aoc5-

Twin Cities Gay Mommies: https://www.facebook.com/groups
/177929668979444/

Mississippi

Gulf Coast Equality Counsel: https://www.gulfcoastequality
council.org

Missouri

Kansas City Center for Inclusion: https://www.inclusivekc.org

The GLO Center: https://www.glocenter.org

The Center Project: https://centerproject.org

Montana

The Center—Western Montana's LGBTQ+ Community Center:
https://www.gaymontana.org

Nebraska

Panhandle Equality: http://www.panhandleequality.org/

Out Nebraska: https://outnebraska.org

Nevada

The Center Las Vegas: https://thecenterlv.org/our-programs
/#community

Greater Reno Nevada LGBT Parents: https://www.facebook.com
/groups/281357878721581/

Our Center Reno: https://ourcenterreno.org/programs/

New Hampshire

Seacoast Outright: https://www.seacoastoutright.org

New Jersey

New Jersey Gay Dads: https://www.facebook.com/groups
/742866766118359

Newark LGBTQ Center: https://www.newarklgbtqcenter.org

Hudson Pride Connections Center: https://hudsonpride.org/

The Pride Center of New Jersey, Inc.: http://www.pridecenter.org

Jersey Shore Community Center Project: http://www.jsqspot.org
/index.html

New Mexico

Common Bond: https://www.commonbondnm.org/community
-resources.html

Transgender Resource Center of New Mexico: https://tgrcnm
.org

New York

Pride Center of Western New York: http://www.pridecenterwny
.org/WhoWeAre/AboutUs

Pride and Joy Families / Lesbian and Gay Family Building
Project: http://www.prideandjoyfamilies.org

Hudson Valley LGBTQ Community Center: https://www.lgbtq
center.org

Pride Center of Staten Island: https://www.pridecentersi.org

The Lesbian, Gay, Bisexual & Transgender Community Center:
https://www.gaycenter.org

LGBT Network Center Family Project: https://www.lgbt
network.org

Brooklyn Community Pride Center: www.lgbtbrooklyn.org/

The Loft: www.loftgaycenter.org

The Pride Center of the Capital Region: www.capitalpridecenter
.org

Long Island GLBT Community Center: www.liglbtcenter.org

Central New York Pride: www.cnypride.com

North Carolina

LGBT Center of Raleigh: https://www.lgbtcenterofraleigh.com

LGBT Center of Durham: https://www.lgbtqcenterofdurham.org

Y'all Means All Family Ball: https://www.facebook.com/groups
/566084193944272

Blue Ridge Pride Center: https://blueridgepride.org

Onslow County LGBTQ+ Community Center: https://www.on
slowcountylgbtq.com

North Star LGBTQ Community Center: https://www.northstar
lgbtcc.com

North Dakota

Dakota OutRight: https://dakotaoutright.org

Pride Collective and Community Center: https://www.fmpride
collective.org

Ohio

Family Pride Network of Central Ohio: https://www.familypride
network.org

Gay & Lesbian Community Center of Greater Cincinnati: www
.cincinnatipride.org

The Lesbian, Gay, Bisexual, Transgender Community Center of
Greater Cleveland: www.lgbtcleveland.org

Stonewall Columbus: www.stonewallcolumbus.org/

CANAPI / Akron Pride Center: www.canapi.org

The Greater Dayton LGBT Center: www.daytonlgbtcenter.org/

Full Spectrum Community Outreach: https://www.full
spectrumcommunityoutreach.org

Oklahoma

Enid LGBTQ: https://www.enidlgbtq.org

Oklahomans for Equality: https://www.okeq.org

Oregon

Queer Parents of Portland: https://qpoppdx.tumblr.com

Q Center: https://www.pdxqcenter.org

LGBTQ Families of Eugene: https://www.facebook.com/groups
/LGBTQFamilliesofEugene

Lower Columbia Q Center: https://www.lowercolumbiaqcenter
.org

Pennsylvania

Families Like Ours—LGBTQI Parents in Pittsburgh: https://
familieslikeourspittsburgh.weebly.com

Centre LGBTQA Support Network: https://www.centrelgbtqa
.org

Philadelphia Family Pride: https://www.philadelphiafamilypride
.org

PGH Equality Center: https://pghequalitycenter.org

LGBT Community Center of Central PA: www.central
palgbtcenter.org

William Way LGBT Community Center: www.waygay.org

Gay & Lesbian Community Center of Pittsburgh: www.glccpgh
.org

Common Roads / LGBT Community Center Coalition of
Central Pennsylvania: www.centralpalgbtcenter.org

Lancaster LGBTQ Coalition: https://www.lgbtlancaster.org

LGBTQ Center of Reading: https://www.lgbtcenterofreading
.com

Rhode Island

Rhode Island Pride: https://prideri.org

South Carolina

Parents Night OUT—Harriet Hancock Center: http://
harriethancockcenter.org/parents-night-out/

SC Equality: https://www.scequality.org

Pride Link: https://pridelink.org

South Dakota

Black Hills Center for Equality: http://www.bhcfe.org

Tennessee

Pride Community Center of the Tri Cities: https://pridetricities
.com

Out Memphis: https://www.outmemphis.org

Texas

Borderland Rainbow: https://www.borderlandrainbow.org

Rainbow Roundup: https://www.rrup.org

LGBTQ+ Parents of North Austin: https://www.facebook.com
/groups/425531398038628/

Houston Gay and Lesbian Parents: https://www.facebook.com
/groups/228411994187/

Coastal Bend Pride Center: https://cbpridecenter.org

296   Appendix

Allgo: https://allgo.org/#

Tyler Area Gays: https://tylerareagays.com

Utah

Utah Pride Center: https://utahpridecenter.org/

Vermont

Outright Vermont: https://www.outrightvt.org

Pride Center Vermont: https://www.pridecentervt.org

Virginia

Diversity Richmond: https://www.diversityrichmond.org

LGBT Life Center: https://lgbtlifecenter.org

Shenandoah Valley Equality: https://www.svgla.org

Washington

Families of Color Seattle: https://www.focseattle.org/

Puget Sound Queer Families: https://www.rainbowcntr.org/
puget-sound-queer-families *or* https://www.facebook.com
/groups/309961496081945/

Rainbow Center: https://www.rainbowcntr.org/

Gay City: https://www.gaycity.org

Spectrum Resource Center: https://www.spectrumresource
center.org

Rainbow Advocacy Inclusion & Networking Services: https://
www.facebook.com/rains.wa.us

Washington, DC

Rainbow Families: https://www.rainbowfamilies.org

Washington DC Center for GLBT People: http://www.thedc
center.org

West Virginia

West Virginia Gay and Lesbian Community Center: https://
www.facebook.com/wvglcc/

Beckley WV Pride: https://www.beckleypride.org

Wisconsin

Milwaukee LGBT Community Center: https://www.mkelgbt.org

7 Rivers LGBTQ Connect: https://www.7riverslgbtq.org

Outreach LGBTQ+ Center: https://www.outreachmadisonlgbt
.org

LGBT Community Center of the Chippewa Valley: https://www
.cvlgbt.info/

Miltown LGBT Families: http://www.miltownfamilies.org

The LGBT Center of SE Wisconsin: https://lgbtsewi.org

Wyoming

Wyoming Equality: https://www.wyomingequality.org/lgbtq
-resource-guide

Online Community Spaces

Spaces for Solo Parents

http://www.choicemoms.org

https://www.singlemothersbychoice.org

Reddit: r/SingleMothersbyChoice

Facebook

IVF/IUI Single Moms By Choice: https://www.facebook.com
/groups/2055298827850354/about/

Young Single Mothers by Choice: https://www.facebook.com
/groups/1870246909953027/about/

Mocha SMCs: https://www.facebook.com/groups/213829221
9782958/about/

Single Mothers By Choice: https://www.facebook.com/groups
/singlemothersbychoice

Single Mothers by Choice Tryers (SMC TTC): https://www
.facebook.com/groups/SMCttc

Single Mothers By Choice Home Insemination with a Known
Donor https://www.facebook.com/groups/518156955192881

Spaces for LGBTQ+ Families

https://www.queerbirthproject.org
https://www.gayswithkids.com/being
https://rainbowfamilies.org
https://www.familyequality.org
https://loveoverfearwellness.com

Facebook

LGBTQ+ Pregnancy to Parenting

Birthing and Breast or Chestfeeding Trans People and Allies

My Fertility Coach (LGBTQ and TTC)

Queer Parents

LGBTQ+ Pregnancy to Parenthood

Trans/Nonbinary Folks TTC Right Now*

Birthing & nursing masculine of centre #guyslikeus only space
no allies*

Birthing Beyond the Binary

Transfeminine Breastfeeding and Lactation

Mx Seahorse (for updated groups)

Nonbinary parents*

Birthing and Breast and Chestfeeding Trans People and Allies

Trans and Queer Pregnancy and Parenting Group

Bodily Autonomy, Birth Justice, and Infant Feeding

Queer Parents Network

Trans Disabled Parents

Transgender & Non-binary Home-birthing

FTM Dads

Non-binary Pregnancy and Parenting Support

Rad Nonbinary Parents!

Groups with a * are private and closed to cis people. To connect with private Facebook community, join Birthing and Breast or Chestfeeding Trans People and Allies.

Resources for Donor-Conceived People

Donor Conception Network: https://www.dcnetwork.org

Instagram

@donorconceived101

@katie.eggy_conceived

@laurahigh5

Resources for People Experiencing Miscarriage

Pregnancy and Infant Loss Support Centre: https://pilsc.org/

https://www.miscarriagehurts.com

https://thelegacyofleo.com/lgbt-baby-loss/

Partners Too: http://www.miscarriageassociation.org.uk
    /wp-content/
    uploads/2016/10/44051_MA_PartnersToo527_v2.pdf

https://pregnancyafterlosssupport.org/resources-for-lgbtq
    -families-experiencing-loss-and-pregnancy-after-loss/

https://www.emptycradle.org

Recommended Further Reading

Below are other books that explore fertility, solo parenthood, and queer families, for grown-ups and for kids. Links to these books and others, as well as where to buy them, are available on our website, www.babymakingforeverybody.com.

LGBTQ+ Focus

Confessions of Another Mother: Nonbiological Lesbian Moms Tell All by Harlyn Aizley

If These Ovaries Could Talk by Jaimie Kelton and Robin Hopkins

Queer Conception by Kristin Kali

Rad Dad: Dispatches from the Frontiers of Fatherhood by Tomas Moniz and Jeremy Adam Smith

Swelling with Pride: Queer Conception and Adoption Stories by Sara Grafe

Pregnant Butch: Nine Long Months Spent in Drag by A. K. Summers

The Liminal Chrysalis: Imagining Reproduction and Parenting Futures Beyond the Binary, edited by Kori Doty and A. J. Lowik

Journey to Same Sex Parenthood by Eric Rosswood

Does This Baby Make Me Look Straight? Confessions of a Gay Dad by Dan Bucatinsky

And Baby Makes More: Known Donor, Queer Parents & Our Unexpected Families, edited by Susan Goldberg and Chloe Brushwood Rose

Three Dads and a Baby by Ian Jenkins

Reproductive Losses: Challenges to LGBTQ Family-Making by Christa Craven

Solo Parent Focus

Single Mothers by Choice: A Guidebook for Women Who Are Considering or Have Chosen Motherhood by Jane Mattes LCSW

An Excellent Choice: Panic and Joy on My Solo Path to Motherhood by Emma Brockes

Going Solo: My Choice to Become a Single Mother Using a Donor by Genevieve Roberts

Choosing Single Motherhood: The Thinking Women's Guide by Mikki Morrisette

Fertility and Cycle-Tracking Focus

Taking Charge of Your Fertility by Toni Weschler

It Starts with an Egg: How the Science of Egg Quality Can Help You Get Pregnant Naturally, Prevent Miscarriage, and Improve Your Odds in IVF by Rebecca Fett

The Fifth Vital Sign by Lisa Hendrickson Jack-Justisse

Period Repair Manual by Lara Briden

Children's Books

What Makes a Baby by Cory Silverberg

The GayBCs by M. L. Webb

Zak's Safari by Christy Tyner

Mommy, Mama, and Me by Lesléa Newman

Two Dads: A Book About Adoption by Carolyn Robertson and Sophie Humphreys

For Mommy So Loved You by Leigh James

Old Enough to Save the Planet by Loll Kirby

We Are Water Protectors by Carole Lindstrom

Notes

Chapter 1

1. Vandenberg-Daves J (nd). Twentieth-Century American Motherhood: Promises, Pitfalls, and Continuing Legacies. *The American Historian* (Organization of American Historians). https://www.oah.org/tah/issues/2016/november/twentieth-century-american-motherhood-promises-pitfalls-and-continuing-legacies.

2. The Lesbian Mothers National Defense Fund (LMNDF) (nd). *Outhistory*. Retrieved June 30, 2022, from https://outhistory.org/exhibits/show/lmndf/lmndf; Rudolph D (2017, October 20). A Very Brief History of LGBTQ Parenting. *Family Equality* (blog). Retrieved June 30, 2022, from https://www.familyequality.org/2017/10/20/a-very-brief-history-of-lgbtq-parenting.

3. Family Equality Council (2019, January). LGBTQ Family Building Survey Executive Summary. *Family Equality* (blog). https://www.familyequality.org/resources/lgbtq-family-building-survey.

4. Single Parents by Choice (nd). Reproductive Science Center. https://rscbayarea.com/treatments/single-mothers-by-choice.

5. Maintaining Connections with Birth Families in Adoption (nd). Child Welfare Information Gateway. https://www.childwelfare.gov/topics/adoption/preplacement/adoption-openness.

Chapter 2

1. Goleman D (1986, December 2). Major Personality Study Finds That Traits Are Mostly Inherited. *New York Times*. https://www.nytimes.com/1986/12/02/science/major-personality-study-finds-that-traits-are-mostly-inherited.html.

2. Hatem A (2020, September 17). Sperm Donors Are Almost Always White, and It's Pushing Black Parents Using IVF to Start Families That Don't Look Like Them. *Insider*. https://www.insider.com/egg-sperm-donor-diversity-lacking-race-2020-9; US Food and Drug Administration (2018, March 22). Donor Eligibility Final Rule and Guidance Question and Answers. USFDA. https://www.fda.gov/vaccines-blood-biologics/tissue-tissue-products/donor-eligibility-final-rule-and-guidance-questions-and-answers.

3. Ishii T, de Miguel Beriain I (2022). Shifting to a Model of Donor Conception That Entails a Communication Agreement Among the Parents, Donor,

and Offspring. *BMC Medical Ethics* 23(18). https://doi.org/10.1186/s12910-022 -00756-1.

4. Fertility and Ovulation (nd). Sperm Bank of California. Retrieved June 30, 2022, from https://www.thespermbankofca.org/fertility-and-ovulation.

5. Carroll N, Palmer J (2001). A Comparison of Intrauterine Versus Intracervical Insemination in Fertile Single Women. *Fertility and Sterility* 75(4), 656–60. https://doi.org/10.1016/S0015-0282(00)01782-9; Byrd W, Bradshaw K, Carr B, Edman C, Odom J, Ackerman G (1990). A Prospective Randomized Study of Pregnancy Rates Following Intrauterine and Intracervical Insemination Using Frozen Donor Sperm. *Fertility and Sterility* 53(3), 521–27. https://doi .org/10.1016/S0015-0282(16)53351-2.

6. USFDA. Donor Eligibility Final Rule.

7. Gong D, Liu YL, Zheng Z, Tian YF, Li Z (2009). An Overview on Ethical Issues About Sperm Donation. *Asian Journal of Andrology* 11(6), 645–52. https:// doi.org/10.1038/aja.2009.61.

8. Goleman. *Major Personality Study Finds.*

9. Hatem. *Sperm Donors Are Almost Always White.*

10. Vaughn R (2021, March 12). Why Is There a Shortage of Black Egg Donors and Black Sperm Donors? International Fertility Law Group. https://www.iflg .net/black-egg-donor-sperm-donor-shortage; Perez MZ (2018, November 28). Where Are All The Sperm Donors of Color? Rewire News Group. https:// rewirenewsgroup.com/article/2018/11/28/where-are-all-the-sperm-donors -of-color.

11. Ravelingien A, Provoost V, Pennings G (2013). Donor-Conceived Children Looking for Their Sperm Donor: What Do They Want to Know? *Facts, Views & Vision in ObGyn* 5(4), 257–64. https://www.ncbi.nlm.nih.gov/pmc/articles /PMC3987373.

12. Smotrich D, Botes A, Wang X, Gaona M, Batzofin D (2015). Gay Surrogacy— the Quandry [sic] of Accessing Verifiable Facts [Abstract]. *Fertility and Sterility* 104(3), Supplement e33. https://doi.org/10.1016/j.fertnstert.2015.07.101.

13. Centers for Disease Control and Prevention (2021). *2019 Assisted Reproductive Technology Fertility Clinic and National Summary Report.* US Department of Health and Human Services. https://www.cdc.gov/art/reports /2019/pdf/2019-Report-ART-Fertility-Clinic-National-Summary-h.pdf#page =29; Estes M (2016, March 10). Accepting Using a Donor Egg. *Aspire Blog.* Retrieved June 30, 2022, from https://www.aspirefertility.com/blog/accep ting-using-a-donor-egg.

14. Embryo Freezing (nd). Human Fertilisation and Embryology Authority. Retrieved June 30, 2022, from https://www.hfea.gov.uk/treatments/fertility -preservation/embryo-freezing.

15. Hatem. *Sperm Donors Are Almost Always White.*

16. Summers A (2021, May 7). Lack of Minority Egg Donors May Depend on Region and Race. CBS8. https://www.cbs8.com/article/life/family/lack-of

-minority-egg-donors-depend-on-region-and-race/509-29c21537-b39e-412c -af01-45d8c75671e4; Carter B (2020, January 13). Why Can't I Find an Afro-Caribbean Egg Donor? BBC News. https://www.bbc.com/news/stories -51065910.

17. Smotrich et al. Gay Surrogacy.; American Society for Reproductive Medicine (2016). Fact Sheet: Egg Donation. https://www.reproductivefacts.org /globalassets/rf/news-and-publications/bookletsfact-sheets/english-fact -sheets-and-info-booklets/egg_donation_factsheet.pdf; American Society for Reproductive Medicine (2018). Third-Party Reproduction: Sperm, Egg, and Embryo Donation and Surrogacy. https://www.reproductivefacts.org/news -and-publications/patient-fact-sheets-and-booklets/documents/fact-sheets -and-info-booklets/third-party-reproduction-sperm-egg-and-embryo -donation-and-surrogacy.

18. Intended Parents: Egg Donor Fees & Costs (2022, June 18). Egg Donor America, Egg Bank America. Retrieved June 30, 2022, from https://www.egg donoramerica.com/parents/egg-donor-fees-costs.

19. How to Find a Surrogate Mother (2022). American Surrogacy. https://www .americansurrogacy.com/parents/finding-a-surrogate-mother.

20. Leondires MP (2022). How Do I Find a Surrogate? Gay Parents To Be. https:// www.gayparentstobe.com/gay-parenting-blog/how-to-find-a-surrogate.

21. Understanding Surrogacy Costs (2022). Circle Surrogacy and Egg Donation. Retrieved June 30, 2022, from https://www.circlesurrogacy.com/parents /how-it-works/surrogacy-cost; Houghton W (2022). The Surrogacy Guide: The Average Cost of Surrogacy. Sensible Surrogacy. Retrieved June 30, 2022, from https://www.sensiblesurrogacy.com/surrogacy-costs.

22. How Much Does Surrogacy Cost in North Carolina? (2018). Parker Herring Law Group, PLLC. Retrieved June 30, 2022, from https://parkerherring lawgroup.com/surrogacy-lawyer-attorney-raleigh-nc/intended-parents /how-much-does-surrogacy-cost.

Chapter 3

1. Macken J (2017, May 17). How Many Eggs Do I Have? Clear Blue. Retrieved June 30, 2022, from https://www.clearblue.com/how-to-get-pregnant/how -many-eggs-do-i-have.

2. Basal Body Temperature (BBT) Charting (2020, October 8). University of Michigan Health. https://www.uofmhealth.org/health-library/hw20205.

3. Basal Body Temperature (BBT) Charting. https://www.uofmhealth.org/health -library/hw202058.

4. US Department of Health and Human Services (2021, February 22). Polycystic Ovary Syndrome. Office on Women's Health. Retrieved June 30, 2022, from https://www.womenshealth.gov/a-z-topics/polycystic-ovary-syndrome.

5. Agrawal R, Sharma S, Bekir J, Conway G, Bailey J, Balen AH, Prelevic G (2004). Prevalence of Polycystic Ovaries and Polycystic Ovary Syndrome in

Lesbian Women Compared with Heterosexual Women. *Fertility and Sterility* 82(5), 1352–57. https://doi.org/10.1016/j.fertnstert.2004.04.041.

6. Kumar N, Singh AK (2015). Trends of Male Factor Infertility, an Important Cause of Infertility: A Review of Literature. *Journal of Human Reproductive Sciences* 8(4), 191–96. https://doi.org/10.4103/0974-1208.170370.

7. Gaskins AJ, Afeiche MC, Wright DL, Toth TL, Williams PL, Gillman MW, Hauser R, Chavarro JE (2014). Dietary Folate and Reproductive Success Among Women Undergoing Assisted Reproduction. *Obstetrics & Gynecology* 124(4), 801–09. https://doi.org/10.1097/AOG.0000000000000477.

8. Endocrine Today (2010, December 1). Dietary Fats, Fatty Acids Affect Sperm Quality. *Healio*. Retrieved June 30, 2022 from https://www.healio.com/news/endocrinology/20120325/dietary-fats-fatty-acids-affect-sperm-quality.

9. Brown MJ (2020, August 13). 16 Ways to Naturally Boost Fertility. *Healthline*. Retrieved June 30, 2022, from https://www.healthline.com/nutrition/16-fertility-tips-to-get-pregnant#2.-Eat-a-bigger-breakfast.

10. Ding GL, Liu Y, Liu ME, Pan JX, Guo MX, Sheng JZ, Huang HF (2015). The Effects of Diabetes on Male Fertility and Epigenetic Regulation During Spermatogenesis. *Asian Journal of Andrology* 17(6), 948–53. https://doi.org/10.4103/1008-682X.150844.

11. Zhu J, Arsovka B, Kozovska K (2018). Acupuncture Treatment for Fertility. *Open Access Macedonian Journal of Medical Sciences* 6(9), 1685–87. https://doi.org/10.3889/oamjms.2018.379; Acupuncture for Fertility (2021). American Pregnancy Association. Retrieved June 30, 2022, from https://americanpregnancy.org/getting-pregnant/acupuncture-for-fertility.

12. Pinto A (nd). How Hydration Affects Fertility. ReproMed Fertility Center. Retrieved June 30, 2022, from https://www.repromedfertility.com/blog/how-hydration-affects-fertility-4153.

13. Boivin J, Sanders K, Schmidt L (2006). Age and Social Position Moderate the Effect of Stress on Fertility. *Evolution and Human Behavior* 27(5), 345–56. https://doi.org/10.1016/j.evolhumbehav.2006.03.004.

14. Ilacqua A, Izzo G, Emerenziani GP, Baldari C, Aversa A (2018). Lifestyle and Fertility: The Influence of Stress and Quality of Life on Male Fertility. *Reproductive Biology and Endocrinology* 16(1), 115. https://doi.org/10.1186/s12958-018-0436-9.

15. Cornell University (2020, February 25). Spending Time in Nature Reduces Stress. *ScienceDaily*. Retrieved June 30, 2022, from www.sciencedaily.com/releases/2020/02/200225164210.htm.

16. Kubala J (2022, January 20). 16 Ways to Relieve Stress. *Healthline*. Retrieved June 30, 2022, from https://www.healthline.com/nutrition/16-ways-relieve-stress-anxiety#3.-Minimize-phone-use-and-screen-time.

17. Isidori AM, Pozza C, Gianfrilli G, Isidori A (2006). Medical Treatment to Improve Sperm Quality. *Reproductive Biomedicine Online* 12(6), 704–14. https://www.rbmojournal.com/article/S1472-6483(10)61082-6/pdf.

18. Rodriguez H (2021, May 12). Maca, Wonder Herb for Fertility. *Natural Fertility Info*. Retrieved June 30, 2022, from https://natural-fertility-info.com/maca.

19. Daniele C, Thompson Coon J, Pittler MH, Ernst E (2005). *Vitex agnus castus*: A Systematic Review of Adverse Events. *Drug Safety* 28(4), 319–32. https://pubmed.ncbi.nlm.nih.gov/15783241.

20. Florou P, Anagnostis P, Theocharis P, Chourdakis M, Goulis DG (2020). Does Coenzyme Q10 Supplementation Improve Fertility Outcomes in Women Undergoing Assisted Reproductive Technology Procedures? A Systematic Review and Meta-Analysis of Randomized-Controlled Trials. *Journal of Assisted Reproduction and Genetics* 37(10), 2377–87. https://doi.org/10.1007/s10815-020-01906-3.

21. Widra E (2022, January 31). How Vitamin D Affects Your Fertility. Shady Grove Fertility. https://www.shadygrovefertility.com/article/how-vitamin-d-affects-your-fertility.

22. Stanhiser J, Jukic AM, Steiner AZ (2019, September 1). Omega-3 Fatty Acid Supplementation and Fecundability. *Fertility and Sterility* 12(3), Supplement E28. https://doi.org/10.1016/j.fertnstert.2019.07.205.

Chapter 4

1. Artal-Mittelmark R (2021, May). Stages of Development of the Fetus. *Merck Manual Consumer Version*. https://www.merckmanuals.com/home/women-s-health-issues/normal-pregnancy/stages-of-development-of-the-fetus.

2. Corson SL, Batzer FR, Otis C, Fee D (1986, May). The Cervical Cap for Home Artificial Insemination. *Journal of Reproductive Medicine* 31(5): 349–52. PMID: 3746786.

3. https://www.nejm.org/doi/full/10.1056/nejm199512073332301.

4. Muthigi A, Jahandideh S, Bishop LA, Shin P, Devine K, Tanrikut C (2020). Clarifying the Relationship Between Total Motile Sperm Counts (TMSC) and Intrauterine Insemination (IUI) Pregnancy Rates. *Fertility and Sterility* 114(3), Supplement e362. https://doi.org/10.1016/j.fertnstert.2020.08.1078.

5. Di Santo M, Tarozzi N, Nadalini M, Borini A (2012). Human Sperm Cryo-preservation: Update on Techniques, Effect on DNA Integrity, and Implications for ART. *Advances in Urology* 2012, 854837. https://doi.org/10.1155/2012/854837.

6. Kop PA, Mochtar MH, O'Brien PA, Van der Veen F, van Wely M (2018). Intra-uterine Insemination Versus Intracervical Insemination in Donor Sperm Treatment. *Cochrane Database of Systemic Reviews* 1(1). https://doi.org/10.1002/14651858.CD000317.pub4.

7. Custers IM, Flierman PA, Maas P, Cox T, Van Dessel TJHM, Gerards MH, et al. (2009). Immobilisation Versus Immediate Mobilisation After Intrauter-ine Insemination: Randomised Controlled Trial. *BMJ* 339:b4080. doi:10.1136/bmj.b4080. https://www.bmj.com/content/339/bmj.b4080.

8. Philippe M, Heraud MH, Grenier N, Lourdel E, Sanguinet P, Copin H (2010). Predictive Factors for Pregnancy After Intrauterine Insemination (IUI): An Analysis of 1038 Cycles and a Review of the Literature. *Fertility and Sterility* 93(1), 79–88. https://doi.org/10.1016/j.fertnstert.2008.09.058.

9. Kop PA, van Wely M, Mol BW, de Melker AA, Janssens PM, Arends B, Curfs MH, Kortman M, Nap A, Rijnders E, Roovers JP, Ruis H, Simons AH, Repping S, van der Veen F, Mochtar MH (2015). Intrauterine Insemination or Intracervical Insemination with Cryopreserved Donor Sperm in the Natural Cycle: A Cohort Study. *Human Reproduction* 30(3), 603–07. https://doi.org/10.1093/humrep/dev004; Haebe J, Martin J, Tekepety F, Tummon I, Shepherd K (2002). Success of Intrauterine Insemination in Women Aged 40–42 Years. *Fertility and Sterility* 78(1), 29–33. https://doi.org/10.1016/S0015-0282(02)03168-0.

10. Johal J, Gardner R, Vaughn S, Jaswa E, Hedlin H, Aghajanova L (2021). Pregnancy Success Rates for Lesbian Women Undergoing Interauterine Insemination. *Fertility and Sterility* 2(3), 275–81. https://doi.org/10.1016/j.xfre.2021.04.007.

11. Johal et al. Pregnancy Success Rates for Lesbian Women.

12. Kryou D, Riva A, Verpoest W, Fatemi HM, Tournaye H, Devroey P (2010). What Is the Optimal Moment for IUI in Natural Cycles? Human Chorionic Gonadotropin or Luteinizing Monitoring? Preliminary Results of a Randomized Study. *Fertility and Sterility* 94(4), Supplement 170. https://doi.org/10.1016/j.fertnstert.2010.07.674.

13. Simpson S, Pal L (2020). IUI After LH Surge: How Soon Is Too Soon? *Fertility and Sterility* 114(3), Supplement e224. https://doi.org/10.1016/j.fertnstert.2020.08.629.

14. Hill MJ, Richter KS, Zareck SM, DeCherney AH, Osheroff JE, Levens ED (2013). Single and Double Donor Sperm Intrauterine Insemination Cycles for Male Factor Infertility: Does Double IUI Increase Clinical Pregnancy Rates? *Fertility and Sterility* 100(3), Supplement 71. https://doi.org/10.1016/j.fertnstert.2013.07.1900.

15. Monseur BC, Franasiak JM, Sun L, Scott RT Jr., Kaser DJ (2019). Double Intrauterine Insemination (IUI) of No Benefit Over Single IUI Among Lesbian and Single Women Seeking to Conceive. *Journal of Assisted Reproduction and Genetics* 36(10), 2095–101. https://doi.org/10.1007/s10815-019-01561-3.

16. Johal et al. Pregnancy Success Rates for Lesbian Women; Dovey S, Sneeringer RM, Penzias AS (2008). Clomiphene Citrate and Intrauterine Insemination: Analysis of More than 4100 Cycles. *Fertility and Sterility* 90(6), 2281–86. https://doi.org/10.1016/j.fertnstert.2007.10.057.

17. Carpinello OJ, Jahandideh S, Yamasaki M, Hill MJ, Decherney AH, Stentz N, Moon KS, Devine K (2021). Does Ovarian Stimulation Benefit Ovulatory Women Undergoing Therapeutic Donor Insemination? *Fertility and Sterility* 115(3), 638–45. https://doi.org/10.1016/j.fertnstert.2020.08.1430.

18. Nordqvist S, Sydsjo G, Lampic C, Akerud H, Elenis E, Svanberg AS (2014). Sexual Orientation of Women Does Not Affect Outcome of Fertility Treatment with Donated Sperm. *Human Reproduction* 29(4), 704–11. https://doi.org/10.1093/humrep/det445; Soares SR, Cruz M, Vergara V, Requena A, Garcia-Velasco JA (2019). Donor IUI Is Equally Effective for Heterosexual Couples, Single Women and Lesbians, but Autologous IUI Does Worse. *Human Reproduction* 34(11), 2184–92. https://doi.org/10.1093/humrep/dez179.

19. Cohlen B, Bijkerk A, Van der Poel S, Ombelet W (2018). IUI: Review and Systematic Assessment of the Evidence That Supports Global Recommendations. *Human Reproduction Update* 24(3), 300–19. https://doi.org/10.1093/humupd/dmx041.

20. Wan JP, Wang ZJ, Sheng Y, Chen W, Guo QQ, Xu J, Fan HR, Sun M (2020). Effect of HCG-Triggered Ovulation on Pregnancy Outcomes in Intrauterine Insemination: An Analysis of 5,610 First IUI Natural Cycles with Donor Sperm in China. *Frontiers in Endocrinology* 11(423), 1–6. https://doi.org/10.3389/fendo.2020.00423.

21. Santistevan A, Cohn KH, Schnorr J, Copperman AB, Widra EA, Yurttas Beim P (2016). Development of Personalized Predictive Models for Non-IVF and IVF Procedures in Lesbian and Single Women Sheds Light on Applicability of Infertility Biomarkers to Women of Unknown Fertility Status. *Fertility and Sterility* 106(3), Supplement e173. https://doi.org/10.1016/j.fertnstert.2016.07.508.

22. Diego D, Medline A, Katler QS, Hipp HS, Kawwass JF, Chen AH (2021). Fertility Treatment Choices and Pregnancy Outcomes Among Single Lesbian Women. *Fertility and Sterility* 116(3), Supplement e248. https://doi.org/10.1016/j.fertnstert.2021.07.665; Bodri D, Nair S, Gill A, Lamanna G, Rahmati M, Arian-Schad M, Smith V, Linara E, Wang J, Macklon N, Ajuja KK (2018). Shared Motherhood IVF: High Delivery Rates in a Large Study of Treatments for Lesbian Couples Using Partner-Donated Eggs. *Reproductive Biomedicine Online* 36(2), 130–36. https://doi.org/10.1016/j.rbmo.2017.11.006.

23. Centers for Disease Control and Prevention (nd). Assisted Reproductive Technology (ART) Data. Retrieved June 30, 2022, from https://nccd.cdc.gov/drh_art/rdPage.aspx?rdReport=DRH_ART.ClinicInfo&rdRequestForward=True&ClinicId=9999&ShowNational=1.

24. CDC. *2019 Assisted Reproductive Technology.*

Chapter 5

1. Armuand G, Dhejne C, Olofsson JI, Rodriguez-Wallberg KA (2017). Transgender Men's Experiences of Fertility Preservation: A Qualitative Study. *Human Reproduction* 32(2), 383–90. https://doi.org/10.1093/humrep/dew323.

2. World Health Organization (2010). *WHO Laboratory Manual for the Examination and Processing of Human Semen*, 5th ed. https://apps.who.int/iris

/bitstream/handle/10665/44261/9789241547789_eng.pdf;jsessionid=F577E96
867A29CC002AE25F470B4FFF3?sequence=1.

3. Yan M, Bustos SS, Kuruoglu D, Ciudad P, Forte AJ, Kim EA, Del Corral G, Manrique OJ (2021). Systematic Review of Fertility Preservation Options in Transgender Patients: A Guide for Plastic Surgeons. *Annals of Translational Medicine* 9(7), 613. https://doi.org/10.21037/atm-20-4523; Amato P (2016, June 17). Fertility Options for Transgender Persons. UCSF Transgender Care. University of California San Francisco Medical Center. https://transcare.ucsf.edu/guidelines/fertility; Schneider F, Kliesch S, Schlatt S, Neuhaus N (2017). Andrology of Male-to-Female Transsexuals: Influence of Cross-Sex Hormone Therapy on Testicular Function. *Andrology* 5(5), 873–80. https://doi.org/10.1111/andr.12405.

4. Adeleye AJ, Reid G, Kao CN, Mok-Lin E, Smith, JF (2019). Semen Parameters Among Transgender Women with a History of Hormonal Treatment. *Urology* 124, 136–41. https://doi.org/10.1016/j.urology.2018.10.005.

5. Schulze C (1988). Response of the Human Testis to Long-Term Estrogen Treatment: Morphology of Sertoli Cells, Leydig Cells and Spermatogonial Stem Cells. *Cell & Tissue Research* 251, 31–43. https://doi.org/10.1007/BF00215444; Lübbert H, Leo-Rossberg I, Hammerstein J (1992). Effects of Ethinyl Estradiol on Semen Quality and Various Hormonal Parameters in a Eugonadal Male. *Fertility and Sterility* 58(3), 603–608. https://doi.org/10.1016/S0015-0282(16)55271-6.

6. Matoso A, Khandakar B, Yuan S, Wu T, Wang LJ, Lombardo KA, Mangray S, Mannan AASR, Yakirevich E (2018). Spectrum of Findings in Orchiectomy Specimens of Persons Undergoing Gender Confirmation Surgery. *Human Pathology* 76, 91–99. https://doi.org/10.1016/j.humpath.2018.03.007.

7. Hembree WC, Cohen-Kettenis P, Delemarre-van de Waal HA, Gooren LJ, Meyer WJ III, Spack NP, Tangpricha V, Montori VM (2009). Endocrine Treatment of Transsexual Persons: An Endocrine Society Clinical Practice Guideline. *Journal of Clinical Endocrinology & Metabolism* 94(9), 3132–54. https://doi.org/10.1210/jc.2009-0345; Leavy M, Trottmann M, Liedl B, Reese S, Stief C, Freitag B, Baugh J, Spagnoli G, Kolle S (2017). Effects of Elevated β-Estradiol Levels on the Functional Morphology of the Testis—New Insights. *Scientific Reports* 7, 39931. https://doi.org/10.1038/srep39931.

8. de Nie I, Meißner A, Kostelijk EH, Soufan AT, Voorn-de Warem IAC, den Heijer M, Huirne J, van Mello NM (2020, July). Impaired Semen Quality in Trans Women: Prevalence and Determinants. *Human Reproduction* 35(7), 1529–36. https://doi.org/10.1093/humrep/deaa133.

9. de Nie et al. Impaired Semen Quality in Trans Women.

10. Liu PY, Turner L, Rushford D, McDonald J, Baker HW, Conway AJ, Handelsman DJ (1999). Efficacy and Safety of Recombinant Human Follicle Stimulating Hormone (Gonal-F) with Urinary Human Chorionic Gonadotrophin for Induction of Spermatogenesis and Fertility in Gonadotrophin-Deficient

Men. *Human Reproduction* 14(6), 1540–45. https://doi.org/10.1093/humrep/14.6.1540.

11. Goldfarb L, Newman J (2022). The Protocols for Induced Lactation: A Guide for Maximizing Breastmilk Production. Retrieved June 30, 2022, from https://www.asklenore.info/breastfeeding/induced_lactation/protocols4print.shtml.

12. Trautner E, McCool-Myers M, Joyner AB (2020). Knowledge and Practice of Induction of Lactation in Trans Women Among Professionals Working in Trans Health. *International Breastfeeding Journal* 15, 63. https://doi.org/10.1186/s13006-020-00308-6.

13. Sehat B, Demir M, Ozdemir O, Yuksel K (2018). A Meta-Analysis on the Cardiac Safety Profile of Domperidone Compared to Metoclopramide. *United European Gastroenterology Journal* 6(9), 1331–46. https://doi.org/10.1177/2050640618799153.

14. Cunha JP (2022, May 5). Reglan. RxList. Retrieved June 30, 2022, from https://www.rxlist.com/reglan-side-effects-drug-center.htm.

15. Reisman T, Goldstein Z (2018). Case Report: Induced Lactation in a Transgender Woman. *Transgender Health* 3(1). https://doi.org/10.1089/trgh.2017.0044.

16. Lewis R (2019, October 30). Fenugreek for Breastmilk: How This Magical Herb May Help with Supply. *Healthline*. Retrieved June 30, 2022, from https://www.healthline.com/health/breastfeeding/fenugreek-breastfeeding#dose.

17. Mallory J, Martinez S, Shah S (2017, February). Supplement Sampler: Natural Galactagogues. University of Wisconsin Department of Family Medicine and Community Health—Integrative Health. https://www.fammed.wisc.edu/files/webfm-uploads/documents/outreach/im/ss_galactogogues.pdf.

18. Light A, Wang LF, Zeymo A, Gomez-Lobo V (2018). Family Planning and Contraception Use in Transgender Men. *Contraception: An International Reproductive Health Journal* 98(4), 266–69. https://doi.org/10.1016/j.contraception.2018.06.006.

19. Light et al. Family Planning and Contraception Use.

20. Loverro G, Resta L, Dellino M, Edoardo DN, Cascarano MA, Loverro M, Mastrolia SA (2016). Uterine and Ovarian Changes During Testosterone Administration in Young Female-to-Male Transsexuals. *Taiwanese Journal of Obstetrics and Gynecology* 55(5), 686–91. https://doi.org/10.1016/j.tjog.2016.03.004.

21. Leung A, Sakkas D, Pang S, Thornton K, Resetkova N (2019). Assisted Reproductive Technology Outcomes in Female-to-Male Transgender Patients Compared with Cisgender Patients: A New Frontier in Reproductive Medicine. *Fertility and Sterility* 112(5), 858–65. https://doi.org/10.1016/j.fertnstert.2019.07.014.

22. Liu M, Murthi S, Poretsky L (2020). Polycystic Ovary Syndrome and Gender Identity. *Yale Journal of Biology and Medicine* 93(4), 529–37.

23. Besse M, Lampe NM, Mann ES (2020). Experiences with Achieving Pregnancy and Giving Birth Among Transgender Men: A Narrative Literature

Review. *Yale Journal of Biology and Medicine* 93(4), 517–28. https://www.ncbi .nlm.nih.gov/pmc/articles/PMC7513446; Hoffkling A, Obedin-Maliver J, Sevelius J (2017). From Erasure to Opportunity: A Qualitative Study of the Experiences of Transgender Men Around Pregnancy and Recommendations from Providers. *BMC Pregnancy and Childbirth* 17, Supplement 2, 332. https:// doi.org/10.1186/s12884-017-1491-5.

24. Light AD, Obedin-Maliver J, Sevelius JM, Kerns JL (2014). Transgender Men Who Experienced Pregnancy After Female-to-Male Gender Transitioning. *Obstetrics & Gynecology* 124(6), 1120–27. https://doi.org/10.1097/AOG.00000 00000000540.

25. MacDonald TK (2019). Lactation Care for Transgender and Non-Binary Patients: Empowering Clients and Avoiding Aversives. *Journal of Human Lactation* 35(2), 223–26. https://doi.org/10.1177/0890334419830989.

Chapter 6

1. US Adoption Statistics (2022). Adoption Network. Retrieved June 30, 2022, from https://adoptionnetwork.com/adoption-myths-facts/domestic-us-statistics.

2. Dueholm BJ (2020, April 18). How (and Why) to Become a Foster Parent. *New York Times*. https://www.nytimes.com/article/foster-care.html.

3. Rudolph, A Very Brief History of LGBTQ Parenting.

4. Foster and Adoption Laws (2022, June 29). Movement Advancement Project. Retrieved June 30, 2022, from https://www.lgbtmap.org/equality-maps /foster_and_adoption_laws.

Chapter 7

1. Marcin A (2021, August 24). Is Acupuncture Safe While Pregnant? *Healthline*. Retrieved on June 30, 2022, from https://www.healthline.com/health /pregnancy/acupuncture-during-pregnancy.

2. Baby Loss Information and Support (2022). Tommy's: Together for Every Baby. Retrieved June 30, 2022, from https://www.tommys.org/baby-loss -support/miscarriage-information-and-support/miscarriage-statistics.

3. Parrott J, Goldie J (2019). Best Positive Affirmations for Anxiety Relief: Reduce Anxiety with Affirmations. National Road Safety Partnership Program. Retrieved June 30, 2022, from https://www.nrspp.org.au/resources /best-positive-affirmations-for-anxiety-relief.

4. Sharma A, Madaan V, Petty FD (2006). Exercise for Mental Health. *Primary Care Companion to the Journal of Clinical Psychology* 8(2), 106. https://doi.org /10.4088/pcc.v08n0208a.

5. Legal Status of US Midwives (2020). Midwives Alliance of North America. Retrieved June 30, 2022, from https://mana.org/about-midwives/legal-status -of-us-midwives.

6. Abramowicz J. S. (2013). Benefits and risks of ultrasound in pregnancy. *Seminars in perinatology, 37*(5), 295–300. https://doi.org/10.1053/j.semperi.2013

.06.004; Torloni, M.R., Vedmedovska, N., Merialdi, M., Betrán, A.P., Allen, T., González, R. and Platt, L.D. (2009), Safety of ultrasonography in pregnancy: WHO systematic review of the literature and meta-analysis. Ultrasound Obstet Gynecol, 33: 599-608.

7. How Gender Socialization Impacts Your Child (2022). Northwest Primary Care. https://www.nwpc.com/how-gender-socialization-impacts-children.

8. Is It Safe to Have Sex During Pregnancy? (2021, February). American College of Obstetricians and Gynecologists. Retrieved June 30, 2022, from https://www.acog.org/womens-health/experts-and-stories/ask-acog/is-it-safe-to-have-sex-during-pregnancy.

Chapter 8

1. Cohain JS, Buxbaum RE, Mankuta D. Spontaneous first trimester miscarriage rates per woman among parous women with 1 or more pregnancies of 24 weeks or more. *BMC Pregnancy Childbirth.* 2017;17(1):437. doi:10.1186/s12884-017-1620-1; Wilcox AJ, Weinberg CR, O'Connor JF, et al. Incidence of early loss of pregnancy. *N Engl J Med.* 1988;319(4):189-94. doi:10.1056/NEJM198807283190401.

2. Dulay AT (2020, October). Spontaneous Abortion (Miscarriage). *Merck Manual Professional Version.* Retrieved June 30, 2022, from https://www.merckmanuals.com/professional/gynecology-and-obstetrics/abnormalities-of-pregnancy/spontaneous-abortion.

3. Chu JJ, Devall AJ, Leanne EB, Hardy P, Cheed V, Sun Y, Roberts TE, Ogwulu CO, Williams E, Jones LL, Papadopoulos JHLF, Bender-Atik R, Brewin J, Hinshaw K, Choudhary M, Ahmed A, Naftalin J, Nunes N, Oliver A (2020). Mifepristone and Misoprostol Versus Misoprostol Alone for Management of Missed Miscarriage (MifeMiso): A Randomised, Double-Blind, Placebo-Controlled Trial. *Lancet* 396(10253), 770–78. https://doi.org/10.1016/S0140-6736(20)31788-8.

4. Butler C, Kelsberg G, St. Anna L, Crawford P (2005). Clinical Inquiries: How Long Is Expectant Management Safe in First-Trimester Miscarriage? *Journal of Family Practice* 54(10), 889–90. https://pubmed.ncbi.nlm.nih.gov/16202377.

5. American College of Nurse Midwives (2013). Rh-Negative Blood Type and Pregnancy. *Journal of Midwifery and Women's Health* 58(6), 725–26. https://doi.org/10.1111/jmwh.12140.

6. Ferrazzi E, Tiso G, Di Martino D (2020). Folic Acid Versus 5-Methyl Tetrahydrofolate Supplementation in Pregnancy. *European Journal of Obstetrics & Gynecology and Reproductive Biology* 253, 312–19. https://doi.org/10.1016/j.ejogrb.2020.06.012.

7. Servy EJ, Jacquesson-Fournols L, Cohen M, Menezo YJR (2018). MTHFR Isoform Carriers. 5-MTHF (5-Methyl Tetrahydrofolate) vs Folic Acid: A Key to Pregnancy Outcome: A Case Series. *Journal of Assisted Reproduction and Genetics* 35(8), 1431–35. https://doi.org/10.1007/s10815-018-1225-2; Golja MV, Smid

A, Kuzelicki NK, Trontelj J, Gersak K, Mlinaric-Rascan I (2020). Folate Insufficiency Due to MTHFR Deficiency Is Bypassed by 5-Methyltetrahydrofolate. *Journal of Clinical Medicine* 9(9), 2836. https://doi.org/10.3390/jcm9092836.

8. Newhouse L (2021, March 1). *Is Crying Good for You?* Harvard Health Publishing, Harvard Medical School. Retrieved June 30, 2022, from https://www.health.harvard.edu/blog/is-crying-good-for-you-2021030122020.

9. Wang R, Danhof NA, Tjon-Kon-Fat RI, Eijkemans MJC, Bossuyt PMM, Hochtar MH, van der Veen F, Bhattacharya S, Mol BWJ, van Wely M (2019). Interventions for Unexplained Infertility: A Systematic Review and Network Meta-Analysis. *Cochrane Database of Systemic Reviews* 9. https://doi.org/10.1002/14651858.CD012692.pub2.

10. Kumar N, Singh AK (2015). Trends of Male Factor Infertility, an Important Cause of Infertility: A Review of Literature. *Journal of Human Reproductive Sciences* 8(4), 191–96. https://doi.org/10.4103/0974-1208.170370.

11. Kumar et al. Trends of Male Factor Infertility.

12. Holland K (2018, September 29). Oligospermia and Fertility: What You Should Know. *Healthline.* Retrieved June 30, 2022, from https://www.healthline.com/health/mens-health/oligospermia.

13. Marcello C, Alvarenga C, Pagani R. (2013). The Epidemiology and Etiology of Azoospermia. *Clinics* 60, Supplement 1, 15–26. http://dx.doi.org/10.6061/clinics/2013(Sup01)03.

14. Low Sperm Count (2020, October 30). Mayo Clinic. Retrieved June 30, 2022, from https://www.mayoclinic.org/diseases-conditions/low-sperm-count/symptoms-causes/syc-20374585.

15. What Are Some Possible Causes of Male Infertility? (2017, January 31). Eunice Kennedy Shriver National Institute of Child Health and Human Development. Retrieved June 30, 2022, from https://www.nichd.nih.gov/health/topics/infertility/conditioninfo/causes/causes-male.

16. Causes of Infertility (2020, February 18). NHS. Retrieved June 30, 2022, from https://www.nhs.uk/conditions/infertility/causes.

17. PCOS (Polycystic Ovarian Syndrome) and Diabetes (nd). Centers for Disease Control and Prevention. Retrieved June 30, 2022, from https://www.cdc.gov/diabetes/basics/pcos.html.

18. Lutz J (2020, April 4). The Connection Between Thyroid Disorders and Fertility. *EndocrineWeb* (blog). https://www.endocrineweb.com/thyroid-disorders-fertility.

19. Marsh EE, Al-Hendy A, Kappus D, Galitsky A, Stewart EA, Kerolous M (2018). Burden, Prevalence, and Treatment of Uterine Fibroids: A Survey of US Women. *Journal of Women's Health* 27(11), 1359–67. https://doi.org/10.1089/jwh.2018.7076.

20. Bulletti C, De Zeigler D, Polli V (1999). The Role of Leiomyomas in Infertility. *Journal of the American Association of Gynecologic Laparoscopists* 4(6), 441–45. https://doi.org/10.1016/S1074-3804(99)80008-5.

21. Uterine Anomaly (2022). Columbia Doctors. Retrieved June 30, 2022, from https://www.columbiadoctors.org/treatments-conditions/uterine-anomaly.
22. Endometriosis (2021, March 31). World Health Organization. Retrieved June 30, 2022, from https://www.who.int/news-room/fact-sheets/detail/endometriosis.
23. American Society for Reproductive Medicine (revised 2014). Stress and Infertility. Reproductive Facts. https://www.reproductivefacts.org/news-and -publications/patient-fact-sheets-and-booklets/documents/fact-sheets -and-info-booklets/stress-and-infertility.
24. Mayo Clinic (2013, October 14). Infertility and Stress. *Speaking of Health* (blog). Retrieved June 30, 2022, from https://www.mayoclinichealthsystem .org/hometown-health/speaking-of-health/infertility-and-stress.
25. Infertility in Men Diagnosis (nd). UCSF. Retrieved August 10, 2022, from https://www.ucsfhealth.org/conditions/infertility-in-men/diagnosis.

Chapter 9

1. Kraus T (2018, January 16). How Much Does Stepchild Adoption Cost? Step-parent Adoption. Retrieved June 30, 2022, from https://stepparentadoption .com/much-stepchild-adoption-cost; How Much Does Adoption Cost? (nd). Human Rights Campaign. Retrieved June 30, 2022, from https://www.hrc .org/resources/how-much-does-adoption-cost.

APPENDIX

1. Isidori et al. Medical Treatment to Improve Sperm Quality.
2. Gonzales GF (2011, October 2). Ethnobiology and Ethnopharmacology of *Lepidium meyenii* (Maca), a Plant from the Peruvian Highlands. *Evidence-Based Complementary and Alternative Medicine* 2012, 193496. doi: 10.1155/2012/193496.
3. Compton J (2019, December 27). More LGBTQ Millenials Plan to Have Kids Regardless of Income, Survey Finds. NBC News. https://www.nbcnews .com/feature/nbc-out/more-lgbtq-millennials-plan-have-kids-regardless -income-survey-finds-n1107461.

Index

About the Authors

RAY RACHLIN, LM, CPM (they/she), is a midwife and founder of Refuge Midwifery, licensed in the state of New Jersey since 2017. Ray earned their BS in midwifery at Birthingway College of Midwifery in 2016 and is a member of the Queer and Transgender Midwives Association. Ray lives in Philadelphia, Pennsylvania, with her partner and child.

MAREA GOODMAN, LM, CPM (she/her), is a midwife, writer, and founder of Restore Midwifery. She earned her midwifery degree from the National Midwifery Institute and has been licensed by the Medical Board of California since 2015. She lives in Santa Cruz, California, with her three children and her wife, who is also a midwife.